# Trouble in My Head

# Trouble in My Head

## A Young Girl's Fight with Depression

Translated by Lorenza Garcia

### MATHILDE MONAQUE

LONDON

3 5 7 9 10 8 6 4

Published in 2007 by Vermilion, an imprint of Ebury Publishing

Ebury Publishing is a division of the Random House Group

First Published in France by Les Arènes in 2006

Copyright © Les Arènes, Paris 2006
Translation copyright © Lorenza Garcia 2007

The Random House Group Limited Reg. No. 954009

Addresses for companies within the Random House Group can be found at
www.randomhouse.co.uk

A CIP catalogue record for this book
is available from the British Library

The Random House Group Limited supports The Forest Stewardship
Council (FSC), the leading international forest certification organisation.
All our titles that are printed on Greenpeace approved FSC certified paper
carry the FSC logo. Our paper procurement policy can be found at:
www.rbooks.co.uk/environment

Printed in the UK by CPI Cox and Wyman, Reading, RG1 8EX

ISBN 9780091917234

# Contents

*I began writing...*                                    vii

My struggle with depression                              1

Epilogue                                               151

Afterword by Jeanne Siaud-Facchin                      157

About the Author                                       167

I began writing this account a year after my depression, during a study period one evening at boarding school. I had finished my homework and had some time to spare before going back to my room. For the previous few days I had been thinking about writing again – like I used to during my illness. I opened a large, red notebook, and began remembering...

My book is not the product of a therapeutic exercise: I didn't write it for myself, but more as a way of offering hope to others who suffer from depression, to tell them there really is a way out!

Perhaps in writing about my experience my aim was also to shock people by showing them what depression looks like from the inside – it is often necessary to make people look at things otherwise they won't see them.

Just before I started writing I made the acquaintance of Jeanne Siaud-Facchin, a psychologist who would 'follow' my case for the next six months. I owe a great deal to her; she probably knows me better than anyone.

Not long after, I showed her the first dozen or so pages of my manuscript. She encouraged me to continue writing, and each time we met she asked me how my project was going. And so, as the weeks went by, it began taking shape. Later on I sent my manuscript to a publisher in Paris, who, to my amazement, seemed very interested in my story. She asked me to word-process my manuscript, which I did over the course of one weekend, and I forwarded it to her with the following email:

Dear Madam,

I wanted this text to be accessible, alive, and not to read like an obscure, tedious personal history.

Of course I talk about myself a lot. (I don't see how I could avoid it!) But this is also to make my story sound more credible; after all my depression didn't come out of nowhere! And there had to *be* a story or else what interest would it hold for the reader?

To be honest, when I left the hospital I didn't know why I had suffered from a depressive illness, but I did know why I needed to live, and that the state I had been in was dangerous. I think this is where the interest of my story lies, and it is why I focus not only on the state I was in when I arrived in hospital, but on my quest for truth and happiness.

I also wanted to portray accurately and in all its 'crudity' the treatment I was subjected to, by which I mean my isolation and incomprehension; I wanted to show what it was like, to set my sights very high in order to produce something valuable, but above all truthful.

Yours,

Mathilde

*A few weeks later I signed a writer's contract. Guided by my editor's advice I cut, altered and shaped my manuscript...*

*When I added the last full stop, two years had already gone by since I left the hospital.*

# 1

It is evening. I don't remember the date today. The days of the week mean nothing to me. They pass me by like everything else – always in the same places, always at home. I am in a room where other people pass me by. There are seven others: my two brothers, my three sisters, my parents. I see them, but don't imagine I look at them – they don't interest me. And if they bother me by speaking or asking me a question I am the one who passes . . .

I am here. Silent. Thinking nothing. Empty. The phone rings. Mum is going to answer it and tearfully tell someone I don't know, or at any rate who doesn't matter to me, that my condition is deteriorating. Dad will walk over to her and put his arm around her. I will be silent, watching them – unconcerned. They should never have had me.

I barely flinched when the phone rang. I was busy doing nothing. I don't even have thoughts. Mum is still talking. She seems surprised; relieved and sad at the same time. She has come alive again. She hangs up the phone and rushes over to me, but I remain impassive.

'That was Dr C.'

I had already guessed.

'You can go into hospital this evening.'

I had guessed that too, though I wished I hadn't. And I tell my little voice it can't be true: Dr C said there wouldn't be a bed available for at least two weeks, not until the end of November at the earliest.

Mum is excited. She wants me to hurry up, to get dressed and pack my things. I have no desire to – I have no desire for anything. But I obey because I don't feel like resisting. And besides I agreed to go into hospital if they could cure me – I mean if they could help me out of this hell by doing all the work for me. Because I don't have any strength left. I don't have any strength left.

Not tonight. I didn't want to go there tonight. I needed time to prepare. Mum is hurrying me. She is so pleased they have a bed for me. She loves me. Not me. I don't love anyone. It's more convenient. Loving people is tiring. You see, if I loved one person then I would have to love all the others so they wouldn't pester me. But mostly I am indifferent; I couldn't care less whether she loves me or hates me. Depression is a defence against pain.

I stop putting off the inevitable – another decision not made by me – and pack my bag: three pairs of knickers, some socks, a pair of trousers, a jumper, two T-shirts, and my sponge bag. It only takes a minute. I don't even have time to realise what is happening.

I am already being whisked away, alone, in the back of the empty people carrier. The clock says 7.30pm. Mum is quiet, and it is dark outside. Christmas is almost here and the street decorations should be up, but I don't see any. Mum cannot stand being quiet any longer so she tries to reassure me: 'You'll be fine, you'll see. Everything will be all right!'

I am tormented. Firstly because her words have as much effect on me as crumbs of bread scattered on concrete. But mostly I feel afraid because I am no longer in control. I no longer have the right to choose. I have to go into hospital, but I don't want to go. It isn't a game any more. It's for real now. They've decided: hospital or nothing, hospital or death. Right now I prefer death. I don't want to go into hospital because I haven't had a chance to think about what it means, I who used to think so much. I miss those times. But I won't try to get them back. Maybe they will give them back to me at the hospital.

Suddenly we are there. Mum doesn't take the wrong entrance this time like she did when we went for my first appointment with Dr C: the initial contact is always difficult, but once the machine is running nothing can stop it. Everything goes smoothly, like clockwork. Only I resist: I have never felt the weight of inertia as strongly as I did in the car on my way to that hospital.

# 2

It is strange being at this bleak place so late in the evening. I will realise afterwards that nothing about the way things worked here ever made any sense – as if somehow it was necessary for everything to remain a mystery to me. People were admitted and discharged at all hours of the day and night.

It is dark and the streetlights are on. We walk out of the courtyard and into a lift. It makes a noise. Mum is quiet. She is carrying my bag. She always does everything. She never lets me do anything now so I won't get worn out, and I struggle to 'do' things to show I am still as strong. But I am tired of struggling now. Second floor. A horrible door. White. Locked.

Mum presses the buzzer and an auxiliary nurse comes to open the door. We wait briefly in the day room, which serves as a canteen and has a book cabinet and a ping-pong table in it. A girl is sitting alone at a table. A living being in this soulless world. She looks at me and smiles coldly. Then suddenly Dr C appears. She has stayed on the ward to welcome me. Good evening. I have no money and no mobile phone so we go straight to the room. It is white, but pitch black because the lights are out. There are two beds. A girl is asleep in one. The other is for me.

Dr C switches the light on, and I am thrust into another world – the same cold, stark glare as in the canteen.

Reality hits me and suddenly I know. I understand what I couldn't grasp in the car just now. I realise that my so-called 'short stay' will in fact last a whole month. A month is a long time when you are 14. That's 30 days multiplied by 24 hours. Only 43,200 minutes left to go, 2,592,000 seconds – drip, drip, drip.

The girl in the bed complains about the light. Why don't we leave her alone? It 'pisses her off' being 'pissed about' when she's asleep. Even though she wasn't asleep. I notice a football scarf hanging on a peg. Everything distances me from this place.

'I'm sorry, Houda. Mathilde will be sharing your room. She's just going to put her things away, and then we'll turn the light off.'

I begin unpacking, but Mum stops me. She puts her arms round me. I let her. She will be hurt if I don't and then everything will take longer. This might annoy Houda, who is already in a bad mood. And after all she is my mother, she puts up with me so I should accept her wanting to hug me before she leaves. I can see she's upset, and yet in spite of everything relieved.

She goes with Dr C to sign some papers. I quickly empty the contents of my bag into the wardrobe without saying a word. More than anything I want to get away from Houda's probing eyes. She is wide awake now and seems in a better mood.

'What's your name?'

'Mathilde.'

'How old are you?'

'Fourteen and a half.'

'What's that thing on your head?'

'I've got nits. But don't worry, you won't catch them.'

5

(My whole family had them, and I was wearing a plastic cap as a precaution because Dr C didn't appreciate the idea of having them on her ward.)

'Why are you here?'

Important question. But Houda couldn't care less – she doesn't even wait for a reply. In fact, 'Why are you here?' in hospital is equivalent to 'How are you?' for normal people.

'By the way, keep out of my cupboard! And hands off my stuff, yeah?'

I can't argue with that, and I am not nosy so it makes no difference to me. But I am afraid of this girl and I never ask her why she is here, except when I know she is leaving. I suppose she must be disturbed or anti-social or something.

I almost tell her that I am not in the habit of going through other people's stuff, but I don't. I quickly roll my things up in a ball, turn the light out, and leave.

My relief is short-lived as Dr C catches me on her way out of the nurses' station. It is nearly 8pm and the others have already had their supper. She instructs me to go and eat something, and then turns to Mum who smiles at me sadly before leaving. Karim, one of the male auxiliary nurses, takes over from Dr C. He goes to the fridge, and offers me a choice of the other residents' leftovers: beef, ham, pasta, soup, vegetables and some other repulsive things. I give in to pressure, but only accept the soup. I go and sit down at a table opposite the girl I saw when I arrived.

I am not hungry. I don't want to eat, there's no point. To begin with if I stop existing it won't change anything – especially not here in hospital. No one will notice the difference. They will tell people back home. Some will cry and a lot of others will pretend to and offer their 'condolences'. How ridiculous. I can't stand all this hypocrisy. I am surrounded by sheer evil. I don't want anything. Only to be pure like the beautiful, fair princesses in the stories they used to make me read. My spots have gone. My complexion is almost pure, but not quite. I haven't been polluted like other girls for four months now. They seem perfectly happy, they don't realise it's why they are alive. One day they will be mothers, and maybe they will have children like me, who won't be grateful for having been born.

The girl opposite me is called Lætitia. She looks quite healthy for someone in hospital. She tries to talk to me but I don't feel like listening. I don't want to know.

I stare at my bowl of soup. No! I won't eat. Ever. Leave me alone!

Food disgusts me. We eat it, digest it and excrete it. It's worthless. Like me. So I don't need it. I don't want it. I won't be polluted by it. I refuse. It's degrading. I couldn't even eat if I tried. Just looking at that sludge makes me feel sick, smelling that soon-to-be-rotten odour makes me want to be sick or, if I am not too exhausted and weak, to make myself sick.

Also, I am afraid. I am afraid that if I eat anything my thighs will go lumpy and my stomach will swell up. Obesity is death. Not meaning to offend sick people, but I'd rather have the plague than be obese. Then my decomposition could begin – my path to destruction. Annihilation! I want to deny my existence on earth. I don't feel any sympathy for others who suffer from life because they are unconscious. They can't see, they don't realise that everything is pointless: 'Dust you are and to dust you will return.'

7

I am disgusted by this food in front of me, under my nose, going cold, though it's better cold than hot because it doesn't smell so bad. Karim insists I eat more. His voice echoes in my head. Eat! It's the only word that comes out of their mouths, mouths that mince words and meat – mouths that make me want to be sick when I look at them, so I don't look. I look at the table with the soup on it, and the more I smell it, the more I see it, the less I want to eat. I wish I could go far away. Or rather be far away – going requires effort.

You shouldn't tell me to eat you know, Karim. The more you do, the more I'll become accustomed to your voice and the less I'll hear you. I have already stopped listening to you. Why are you pestering me? Don't you know how frail I am? The others are afraid of bumping into me in case I fall over. I already made a huge effort by eating those three spoonfuls. I've only swallowed a few mouthfuls of water in the last three days. That's 'progress'. You look into my downcast eyes but you don't understand. You keep on insisting, you don't understand, me or others like me. Later you'll say how lucky we are to be here: 'It's easy. You don't need to work, just eat, sleep and be looked after by other people!'

Karim gives up. He already knew he would when he offered me the leftovers. He clears the bowl away. I can go now. Back to 'our' room. I feel like a criminal who has been forced to commit a murder. I wasn't strong enough. I weakly gave in and ate. I am becoming more and more polluted.

In the room Houda is pretending to be asleep – maybe all my talking just now bored her. I put my pyjamas on and turn out the light.

She switches her radio on. I can't believe anyone is allowed to listen to rap music so loud this late, but I don't say anything. It is 8.30pm and I feel like going to sleep. I hate rap music. I don't like R&B either – though I prefer it to this.

When I think Houda is sound asleep, I turn the volume down slightly so I can get some rest too. She wakes up with a start! She is furious and glowers at me.

'Don't touch my stuff!' she says, loud and clear.

Of course I back down. I am upset. I don't know what to do. I get into bed and lie there without moving. I apologise and try to explain but she interrupts me, cuts across me. I was wrong, that's all. She'd warned me not to touch her stuff. Infuriated, she goes back to bed, but not before turning the volume up full blast. A nurse comes to put a stop to the din, which they can hear from the office. She asks if I am all right. Houda glares at me. I daren't tell the truth, especially not on my first night. Yes, yes, we're getting along fine. I like the music, it doesn't bother me.

Houda says it 'soothes' her!

The nurse closes the shutters and goes away again. I desperately want to cry, but I stop myself. I don't want Houda to laugh at me. I need to sleep. To take refuge in the nothingness of sleep. I haven't dreamt for a long time, though I used to dream a lot, and think a lot too. This didn't surprise anyone. People don't go to the doctor because they have an imagination. Unless it is filled with visions of death, awash with dark thoughts!

I long to sink into the darkness that shields my eyes when I close them, to shut out the life swarming around me, making my head spin until I feel dizzy, giddy and sick.

Yet I do not want to die. Something I have always believed in says it is not right. I must not kill myself. It is wrong. And so sordid! So base! I would rather be murdered or die of starvation.

No! I hate violence. I loathe it as much as I do that disgusting food. Why do people resort to violence so easily? Maybe it makes them feel alive: they need to kill some poor guy to prove to themselves they exist. It is mindless. And then they end up in prison, like me, where they aren't allowed to live. Or maybe they are just mad. In any case prison won't help them. Or me.

I would like to sleep now. But I am prevented from satisfying this one desire. Is it the irony of fate?

# 3

The following morning, Tuesday, 6am. A nurse bursts into the room. She says her name is Catherine and smiles at me. I emerge from a semi-sleep. She has come to take a blood sample from me. Houda – who couldn't be in a worse mood given the late night – is also awake. Yet, strangely, this unexpected arrival calms her, the bowl and other equipment arouses her curiosity. After Catherine has said good morning and apologised, Houda bombards her with questions about why she's here, why she, Houda, isn't benefiting from this treatment, and finally why the procedure has to be performed so early as it bothers her greatly.

The nurse doesn't seem unduly concerned by this bleary-eyed fury, and answers her questions evasively while she soaks some cotton wool in antiseptic. Under the inquisitive gaze of Houda, who watches her every movement, she takes hold of my arm, wipes it with antiseptic, throws the cotton wool in the bowl, applies the tourniquet, draws the syringe, and finally sticks the needle in.

'Pump your fist!' Catherine tells me, pointing to my hand. It doesn't seem to want to come out. I feel pleased and I tell myself that maybe at last I truly am weak.

I clench and unclench my fist, fast to begin with, then gradually slower.

'Harder!' Catherine insists.

'I can't!' I say, looking her straight in the eye.

I am unable to move my hand at all now! It feels funny and even quite scary for a second. But I tell myself I won't be needing my limb for very much longer anyway as I am going to die soon. Of course I know perfectly well that my arm isn't in any real danger, I just like imagining my imminent end. And it is strange looking at your own hand without being able to move it – like thinking you can move a vase if you stare at it for long enough. It almost feels like someone else's hand I am looking at.

The nurse loosens the tourniquet, and I feel the blood rushing back into my fingers and slight pins and needles in my legs. This time the blood flows more easily into the syringe and the tubes are soon full. Is that all she's taken? Well, at least it's something.

She tidies everything away and leaves. Houda asks a few more pointless questions and we try to go back to sleep.

# 4

Catherine comes back at 8am and opens the shutters. The light suddenly pouring in blinds us. It is impossible to 'rest' any more. So I look through the window at a tiny patch of blue sky. Beneath it are some grey buildings where other patients must be languishing over breakfast. Everyone says it is terrible here at the hospital, but however good or bad it is will never concern me because it is the simple fact of eating breakfast that disgusts me. All language associated with food and eating makes me feel like being sick – with the exception of cutlery. That cold metal mirrors my appearance, my posture, creating a strange sort of complicity between us, and I think that if I had wanted to do it I would have chosen one of those three.

If I happen to see a knife lying on a table I am plagued by horrible visions of it leaping up and stabbing me in the stomach, as if it had a life of its own. The knife saves my honour by cleansing my stomach of the impurities my cowardly mouth has forced it to suffer.

A fork naturally plunges straight into my carotid artery, and when I think about it I can taste blood in my mouth, and my eyes mist over with strange, red tears. I am like the living dead wanting proof of my condition.

As for the spoon I swallow it whole. It sticks in my throat, piercing it from side to side and choking me.

Then, for dramatic effect, it pops its head out and quietly watches me die.

These are my thoughts when I imagine the first meal of the day, which I refuse to go to. I remain on my bed while Houda complies with the nurses' stringent commands.

Without Houda and her music, I am hoping at last to have a moment's peace to look out at the gloomy hospital grounds, but as luck would have it I can hardly see anything from my bed as it is under the window.

A moment later, though, someone comes along to force me to go in to breakfast, and a pointless discussion ends with me being dragged there. As I walk very self-consciously into the canteen, I feel seven pairs of eyes grouped around two tables turn towards me and begin scrutinising me with a curiosity that is apparently unaffected by the frequent arrivals and departures.

Houda stares at me too, but she is the first to look away. No doubt she has already announced my arrival to the others. I also notice Lætitia, the girl from the night before, in the canteen.

I spot the last empty chair and pull it out from under the table and sit down. The others watch my every move while they continue to eat. They are grumpy and half-asleep, and yet strangely I have roused them all from their usual torpor, except for Houda who remains aloof. My sudden death would only have the effect of making her feel important; she could boast afterwards about how she was there. I think the incident with the radio is too fresh in her mind for her even to be remotely friendly towards me. The others in the canteen talk to me readily, without any of the awkwardness normally associated with a new arrival. No doubt this is a common occurrence as the ward only caters for eight adolescents who are in here for 'short' stays averaging two weeks. Lætitia tries to help me find my bearings and warns me against getting my hopes up. I listen to them, but I don't speak. I haven't much to say, and I don't feel like talking about myself. To begin with it is nobody's business, and secondly I am worn out: I am exhausted from being forced to come in here, and I prefer to stay huddled up quietly on my chair. For the time being I just observe.

'What's your name?'

Do I really have to reply? Can't I have some peace?

I was hoping that here in hospital I could at least quietly vegetate without bothering anyone, without someone always trying to shake me out of my lethargy.

'Mathilde.'

'Are you in here for anorexia?'

They couldn't have made me happier if they had tried, but because I don't think I am thin enough the question sounds silly to me.

'No. Depression.'

I can tell by the look on their faces that some of them attribute my unhappiness to true despair, and not just to my feeling lost or sad at being in hospital. Most of the others are already thinking about something else, this being a routine question which doesn't really mean much.

I dodge the other questions they fling at me and the conversation moves on. I still haven't eaten, disgusted by all those mouths chewing or swallowing almost whole that repulsive food.

# 5

8.30am. I have only been here a few minutes when the others start racing off to the showers, the quicker to get that unavoidable and rather unpleasant activity over with. We are not free to relax and take our time because we must be ready by 9.00 in case a hypothetical doctor asks to see us – though when this rare event did happen it was nearer to 10.00. All that waiting around not knowing used to drive me mad.

It is time I stood up as well. There is so little flesh between my bones and the chair that the weight of my body resting on them is beginning to hurt. The same goes for my spine and I am careful not to lean back for fear of hurting that too.

I remember when I ran my hand down my back I could feel each vertebra easily without needing to bend forward. And anyone looking at the back of my neck would see an amazing succession of bumps and hollows that were quite interesting from an anatomical point of view.

I end up following the general movement. I fetch my clothes, towel and sponge bag and stand by the shower door: an indifferent sentry who would allow anyone to pass without protesting. I wait my turn rather than go back to my – 'our' – room, far preferring to stand beside the open window using up energy than to lie sprawled on the bed.

If that window could talk! It would tell of the hours it spent spying on me while with nothing better to do I watched the daily round of domestics pushing the heavy food trolleys across the courtyard. Occasionally I wondered who they were for or what was in them, and I tried to remember the menu from the day before. But mostly these routine comings and goings were only a distant distraction from the extreme emptiness inside my head.

Today, my first day in hospital, I am in shock. I am enduring not learning. I would be exaggerating if I said I feel indifferent to being here. I feel confused. Coming to the hospital was like burying my whole past, everything unrelated to my relentless departure from life (I wish I could bury time too as it is just another burden). But now I am here I find I can't just carry on dying quietly because I don't know, I don't understand, what they are doing with me here.

I let myself go under because I am the only one who realises, who understands. No one else can see that nothing makes any sense, everything is doomed to failure. We are born and live for no reason. The only thing we have any say over is death. Death is the high point of life, its culmination, in every sense.

The world is rotten. People only enjoy vile pleasures: money, drugs, sex and food. I have rejected all that. I – yes, I – will escape from the vicious circle of dependency, of interdependency between human beings, those vile animals who for some unknown reason are born and live and kill each other; who take their dangerous excesses to strange extremes in their desire to outdo one another; who destroy the beauty and purity of nature, which they don't deserve; who act first and then seeing the consequences of their actions go crying to others who despise them, destroy them or imprison them. And when someone emerges from the crowd who makes people think about the true meaning of dignity, purity, life, he or she is quickly silenced; it would be too awkward if the mechanism were exposed – even though later on it might be taken apart and put back together using those same ideas.

Living is pointless. But so is dying. Which is why I haven't killed myself. In spite of the cutlery, and the plunging stairwells, and the sea, and the cars and the pills!

# 6

I must have been waiting at least 10 minutes by the door to the shower room. I am shivering, turning blue. My nails are blue – not purple, blue – the colour of stormy skies. The rest of me is all white – except for my lips, which are slightly purple. Moonface. Moonstruck. Howling. No, not howling. I am worth less than an animal. I don't have their dignity – or their strength. But I really am on another planet, already floating in space, already dead. I look at everything like a ghost condemned to haunt the lives of others. Already on another planet: craters, dark, lifeless, empty. Like my thoughts. And there's no oxygen here either.

The door flies open, and the fury I share a room with emerges. She gives me a look that is hard rather than mean. Her hair is wet and she is clutching her precious towel. I will always think of her in her pyjamas. She got away with keeping them on until late in the morning even though the rules said we had to be washed and dressed by 9am.

I walk into the shower room and find myself in an asymmetrical space with five walls. As you cross the threshold you are immediately struck by a mirror stretching from the basin to the ceiling on the wall opposite. It is so warped it gives you the impression of being at a fairground and I have a job recognising myself in it. In fact, if I wanted to give my little sister a fright I would only need to stand her in front of this scary object. But for now I am the one who has to put up with its eerie presence, though it doesn't make me feel too strange, no more than usual anyway.

The walls are delicately covered in tiles that are grey-green verging on colourless, which have the virtue of making you forget that beyond this hell is a world full of sunshine, green fields and beauty. I still don't understand how they could reserve a place like this for a ward treating adolescents mainly for depression...

It has a gloomy, mournful atmosphere – not too different, I imagine, from what embalming rooms must have been like in the old days. And indeed, this is the place where future corpses are washed. Have a nice morning!

I brush my teeth. I no longer feel like resisting, and I let my limbs undress me. Ghostlike, I pick up the shower gel from the edge of the basin and I glance at myself in the mirror. I couldn't help it; it haunts the room with its presence.

Then suddenly the mirror has disappeared and I am standing in front of myself, naked. And even if it wasn't warped it would make no difference, I would still be a skeleton.

I see a girl. The same height as me. This bad lighting doesn't flatter her but I don't care. What I am looking at are her bones. There is some skin on them, but not much. I can see my ribcage and the bones in my chest, pelvis and legs. I turn my body round. It's incredible. All my vertebrae are sticking out, as well as my shoulder blades and pelvis. I am fascinated, and a little afraid of this precious living–dying thing at arm's length, within arm's reach. And yet I marvel at it, oblivious. I have never studied anatomy, but I contemplate this living skeleton like a scientist, moving my limbs slowly so I can see the joints working. I slide my hand over my legs. It's amazing how easily I can make my fingers and thumbs meet round my thigh.

I suddenly remember where I am; I don't have all morning and there are others waiting in the queue. I grab the shower gel again and take a last look in the mirror to remind myself I haven't been dreaming, and I step into the shower.

The shower. A white square of sloping tiles with a hole in the middle for the water to drain through. Slippery. You press a button at waist level to make the water come out. I wince as a few thin jets of icy water spurt out and sting me, like in the showers at public swimming pools. The water stops so I press the button again, making sure this time to stand well out of the way.

After several attempts the water finally warms up. I wash, dry myself and get dressed.

# 7

9.30am. Back in my room I tidy my things away and make my bed. Then I head for the nurses' station. It is deserted as always, or almost always. I ask the name of the doctor I will be seeing today, and I am told no one has asked to see me. I return to my room frustrated, my enthusiasm and my eagerness to get better trampled on. I might as well have stayed at home crying in my room. It would have been cheaper for my parents. I hate being a burden.

I lie down on my bed. Houda isn't here. She must be in the TV room. It is cold but I don't feel cold. I never feel cold – even though I don't wear a jumper like everyone else here: I burn up more calories that way – like when I stand.

And I start thinking. There is nothing I can do to escape from this isolation. The people at the hospital don't want to see me. In fact, no one wants to see me, which is why they put me in here in the first place: 'Take her, cure her or just keep her.' She's not good enough! Although she tries to be good, or rather she used to try.

Do you remember how lonely I was during the summer holidays after I caught glandular fever, that stupid illness that leaves you exhausted for up to three months? I didn't see anyone because all my friends had moved away, and it was so sweltering everyone preferred to stay by themselves – even in the house. I was too worn out to do anything but lie in the deck-chair, and the slightest effort made me want to cry. The weather was on my side, though. There was a heatwave.

If only I had caught glandular fever from a kiss! But no. No one cares for me in that way. I am not good enough even for that. It was my brother the champion splutterer who infected me...

It all happened at the beginning of the summer holidays. In early July, my granddad took me and my younger sister Marion with him on his annual walk. This generally consists of a week-long hike in some faraway place, the idea being to familiarise his grandchildren with French, or family history. Granddad has devoted many years to the study of genealogy and after long and painstaking research has accurately traced our family tree back to the time of the French Revolution.

Family history walks consist of stopping at some remote spot near a bend in the path to study a small, precariously balanced pile of stones that looks certain to topple over before the arrival of the next generation, who will have to make do with the photos and accounts of their elders...

Marion and I were treated to a trip to Javols, the old Roman capital of the Lozère region. With all due respect to enthusiasts there was not a lot to see in the tiny museum. As for the amphitheatre, it required a fertile imagination rather than good eyesight to be able to make it out against the landscape, which was very pretty even so!

And so we walked, my indomitable grandfather leading the way intrepidly at the head of the group, while Marion and I struggled to bring up the rear. I was worn out and had to will myself to put one foot in front of the other. I welcomed every break and even cried because I couldn't go on. I longed for my bed. Marion and I managed to persuade our grandfather to alternate walking days with visiting days. Even so, I was still exhausted when I arrived home only to discover that my brother had glandular fever and, given my extreme state of fatigue, I probably did too. I wasn't exactly thrilled by his timing! He could have bothered to be diagnosed sooner and spared me the added exhaustion!

I spent the rest of the holidays lying down. Too tired to read, too tiring to invite anyone round – that is, if there had been anyone to invite. I occasionally managed to slide into the inflatable tub that served as a swimming pool. I ate very little as none of these activities used up much energy.

My loneliness continued even after the beginning of the new school term. My friends had moved to Paris or to Guadeloupe, and I was all by myself at the school opposite our house. I became a recluse, almost never going out. I wrote letters to friends saying I was fine, and that I liked my new class. They were empty words. In a way I was deceiving myself, and yet I knew I had no choice. It was too painful for me to talk about how lonely I was. And anyway people who are alone have nothing to say, and I simply wouldn't have written. The previous year I had fallen out with the only friend I had left. I think we were too close. People sometimes mistook us for twins, and we even unconsciously copied each other's gestures. I think we idealised each other too, and the day we quarrelled it felt as if the world had come to an end. We both suffered a lot and we haven't spoken since. My 'acquaintances' in other classes didn't care about me and I began, inevitably, to flounder. I wasn't the type to cry for help and the few times I tried I was told, 'you'll get over it.'

All of a sudden a man knocks on the door. He has come to show me tomorrow's menu. Caught up in my own thoughts and hardly interested in food I shan't be eating, I mechanically agree to everything. Apparently this routine takes place every morning. Is anything here not a routine? Everything seems very regimented – with little room for variation. Later on Karim will go round with the mop, another daily routine.

Where was I? Oh yes, back at school. I was run down. I had started eating less during the summer because of the heatwave. By the beginning of term I hadn't resumed my normal pattern of eating, and I burnt out at school: you can't function without energy, and energy comes from food. As a lot of doctors and other people were fond of telling me, 'A car can't run without petrol.' This expression used to irritate me intensely: they were criticising my stance (of not eating), which in my quest for perfection was becoming increasingly rigorous, but most of all I found the way they endlessly repeated this phrase patronising.

As a result I stopped listening to everything else they said, and I practised even less what they preached. The only doctor I did listen to evoked the image of a ship without fuel. Also, he let me talk without interrupting and responded to what I said, unlike most of the others who just nodded and changed the subject. The only solution they could think of – besides anti-depressants – was to say, 'Let it all out. Go on, let it all out.' But what was I supposed to be letting out? I wasn't possessed, for goodness' sake!

I tried eating normally but my digestive system had been affected and my metabolism was all messed up. I wasn't used to eating that much food; it gave me terrible stomach aches, and I had to make myself sick in order to ease the pain. Mum overheard me once and dragged me off to see the doctor. All I remember about her was that she had repeated her first year at medical school and she said I had a lot of stretch marks. She made me promise not to make myself sick any more. I began eating even less – it wasn't exactly pleasant being sick anyway.

It became quite normal for me to burst into tears in class, and it reached the point where I was spending whole days in the sick bay: a sick bay with no nurse, just stacks of medicines past their use-by dates, shelves, cupboards, discarded scales and height measures and two uncomfortable looking beds in the next room. I know every centimetre of the *Little Mermaid* and *Aladdin* posters that watched over me blankly during those long weeks.

In the end I stopped going to school completely. The fact is I had pushed myself too hard at the beginning of term to try to compensate for my loneliness. I was top of the class with an average of 18 out of 20, and at home I did all the housework I could to make life easier for the others and to keep myself busy.

What had once been simple tasks now became part of my ideal of perfection. I did everything I was asked, and pre-empted other people's wishes. I felt my presence was distasteful to people and I tried to make them forgive me by being helpful; if I hadn't been such a bore I would have had friends, wouldn't I? Above all I didn't want to be a burden on anyone and I tried my best to make myself small, and to be as good as I could by depriving myself of food, the enemy of purity. But I only succeeded in exhausting myself even more and being less able to do good. I spoke very little. And when I did share my thoughts people would say, 'No. You're wrong.' So I kept quiet. The truth was too blindingly obvious for them to see.

As time went by people began giving me increasingly pained looks, as if I were a poor bird with its wings cut off, bleeding to death. There's nothing we can do, it'll just die. So they look at me blankly, no doubt thinking that will help!

I felt like saying, Stop looking at me like that! Can't you see I'm drowning? Why not throw me a lifebelt instead of just staring at me?

Or you would talk amongst yourselves, casting discreet, pitiful glances at me whenever my name was mentioned.

That didn't help.

I kept thinking, You turn away and laugh amongst yourselves; you are so smug in your contentment, which I don't share because I have replaced it with truth. Why do you never look at me when you're laughing? Are you afraid I'll spoil your fun? Do you despise me? Are you ignoring me?

You know, maybe if you had looked at me and smiled more often (not laughed because then I would have mistrusted you and closed my shell before you had time to see the pearl hidden inside) I might have believed you when you said that life was beautiful...

# 8

A nurse arrives, cutting short my reverie. Her name is Brigitte. She is blonde and looks as though she feels sorry for us because we are in hospital. 'Have you had your shower?' She has come to check my hair for nits. She has a good look and decides that the treatment has been successful. I just have a bit of dandruff, no doubt because I'm run down. Luckily I've got short hair as it's easier with nits. Six days ago I had long hair. It didn't suit me any more so I had it cut. I am even uglier now...

'Where are the others?'

'They've gone for a walk on the beach. Every Tuesday morning there's a walk so you can all get out and stretch your legs.'

'Why didn't anyone ask me if I wanted to go?'

'Because you were in your room. And anyway, you're not strong enough. You haven't eaten anything. We don't want your blood sugar dropping now, do we?'

She goes and fetches a piece of paper, and hands it to me. It is a list of the hospital rules and timetables: timetables and restrictions. I am not allowed to call or receive calls or letters for the first 48 hours. It makes no difference to me, I don't really feel like talking. I tried too hard, and failed.

Brigitte goes out, leaving a handful of lank hairs behind on my brush...

Do you remember the autumn half-term? I had been away from school for a week or two by then. The previous half-term a friend and I had spent writing up a 250-page dissertation entitled 'Youth in the French Resistance'. It was for a competition and the prize was a three-day trip to Alsace with the departmental council. So that autumn I went off on a coach to visit a Nazi concentration camp in Natzweiler-Struthof. It snowed that year. We weren't expecting it to be so cold after such a hot summer and had only brought thin clothes with us. We visited the camp, the rooms where they tortured and dissected people, and the gas chamber – all covered in a layer of glassy ice. It was sinister. We couldn't see more than 3 metres ahead of us in the falling snow and were only just able to make out the huts. We were so cold our minute's silence lasted less than 30 seconds.

It was almost with a feeling of relief that we made our way towards the sheer horrors on show in the museum. Lost in that world of terror far from the towns in the valley below, we felt a little like prisoners ourselves in that strange camp surrounded by trees and impenetrable whiteness. We were glad to climb back on board the warm coach. And do you remember the boarding house we stayed at? They gave us good, hearty, mountain food to warm us up. Everyone seemed to enjoy it thoroughly. Everyone except me...

When I arrived home Mum was preparing to go on a pilgrimage to Medjugorje – a village in Bosnia where the Virgin Mary has been appearing for the last twenty years or more. My brother Maxime wasn't in very good shape at the time, and Mum wanted to entrust him to Mary. When I came back from Struthof she immediately realised I wouldn't be going back to school and she dragged me off with them on another strange adventure. I was to have spent almost my entire holiday sitting on a coach as it took 30 hours by road to reach the remote mountain village. I watched the trees flash by outside the window, and they reminded me of the ones I had just seen in the Black Forest. I watched Mum eating sweets with my brother and a friend of hers. The coachload of elderly people sang canticles for us out of tune. Even such a show of religious devotion did not move me. Finally the people sitting next to me managed to persuade me to take over the microphone from the man in charge, who alone out of all the pensioners deserved first prize for singing off key... In Medjugorje I instinctively retreated to the bathroom to take a relaxing hot shower. But the water went as cold as the room temperature as soon as my hair was wet and I finished rinsing it with cries and chattering of teeth... I went home feeling even weaker than when I had left.

Mum made an appointment with Dr C. I had to tell her about my life, and my present state. 'Do you know the name for what is happening to you?' Of course it had occurred to me but I was afraid of being suddenly alone and having to face reality because it meant going into hospital. 'A depressive disorder.'

Dr C asked me my height and weight, and while she was making a quick calculation I looked at the Anne Geddes photos and strange *The Earth From the Air*-type landscapes on the walls. I found all this soft sentimentality sickening. It didn't go with her cold eyes. 'Your Body Mass Index is 13. We hospitalise at 17 and below.'

So it was true, I had achieved thinness – sort of, anyway. Maybe they would put me on a drip. I wanted to go the whole way before dying. The problem was if they put me on a drip I would gain weight, and I didn't want that. My flesh had to waste away slowly and then I would die. I had no desire to find myself in hospital from one day to the next. I needed to be able to think about it, to control everything.

Dr C was a petite woman with very pale skin, big hazel eyes and light blonde curly hair. She had a pretty, high voice that only ever uttered discouraging words. Her restless, staring eyes were as disturbing as her non-existent smile. She exuded coldness from every pore, and radiated a feeling of discomfort and indifference with regard to us, her poor patients, as if somehow her excessively pale beauty and coldness placed her high above us on a pedestal, inaccessible. In the end we were only her patients, and Dr C wasn't obliged to stick her neck out where we were concerned or even to sympathise with us. She certainly didn't understand us; she was a good scientist of the old school who knew her subject well and was just doing her job. Karim admired her and often said how capable she was – she and another woman doctor who worked on the ward. And yet, although they insist they 'don't discharge you because you're cured, but because you're on the right track', I only ever saw one girl leave the hospital in a good state, and one boy who wasn't in such a bad state when he arrived. On the other hand another girl, Fleur, had been in there once and was back again.

Dr C looks at me with her big, vacant eyes, like a toad's. From then on I decided to think of her as Dr Crapaud.[1]

---

[1] 'Crapaud' is the French word for 'toad'.

Dr Crapaud opens her mouth very slightly – as she has a habit of doing – and tells me there won't be any beds available for two weeks, but that I shall certainly need hospitalising as a matter of urgency.

I was so happy that Friday, thinking that I had time to prepare. What I did not know was that the same time the following Monday they would call to say a bed had miraculously become available and they were expecting me at the hospital.

# 9

11.00. I am all alone in this empty, white room. There is some writing on the walls. I don't remember what it says. I don't care. Time drags on. A minute can last an eternity. I have nothing to do. I have decided to drop everything the way everyone has dropped me – school, activities, everything. Apparently this is a good thing. It will allow me to think about the causes of my depression. As if I hadn't already! It doesn't do any good. Everything eludes me. I can't get a grip on anything. My thoughts spread, fluid and penetrating, into everything around me. It gets me nowhere. My mind is filled with nothingness: a blank, cold vacuum. I am lifeless, responding only with occasional snatches of thought, always angry and frustrated. This doesn't help either. I have had enough of this endless intro–extrospection – of going round in circles.

Does anyone care that my life, my soul, is draining away? The doctors here are paid to look after me, it is their job. But actually they couldn't care less about me. They won't like it if I leave here without being cured because it might harm their reputation. And yet they keep insisting I must cure myself. Maybe I misunderstood: I thought that in hospital they would help me to think, not leave me on my own all day in this big empty room.

# 10

Lunchtime. The others are back with all their troubles in tow: hyperactivity, depression, obese people obsessed by food and family problems...

When I hear them arrive I decide to go to the canteen – there is no point in waiting to be dragged in to lunch. I still feel lost in their company. I feel I belong nowhere.

Karim wheels up the trolley with the food trays. It is a big, box-like object, coloured dark red and cream, that can barely move under its own weight. It gives off an indescribable odour: a mixture of ice-cold starters and puddings, and bland, boiling-hot main courses simmering away and dissolving in their soft, plastic containers swollen by the heat. Everyone takes theirs. Oh look! Mine still has the name of the last person who occupied my bed on it. That's how important I am! In any case I am not hungry.

We sit down to eat and the meal-time ritual begins. Everyone complains about not having got what they asked for and places the unwanted item in the middle of the table for the others to take or for Karim to put back on the trolley. Of course everyone thinks what the person next to them has looks better: they'll choose that tomorrow. In the meantime they swap. Fabien – whose waist is as broad as he is long – ferociously pounces on the discarded first courses exchanging them for his low-cal one, which gets him into trouble with Karim. Mealtimes here are depressing. There isn't any real communication between us. We don't know each other very well, and hardly feel like getting to know each other better while we are eating – an equally unpleasant experience for those accepting this dreadful food as for those refusing it. And then there is Karim constantly looking over our shoulders. And when it isn't him it's one of the nurses…

After they have finished complaining and bickering, they start eating. I don't. The staff take it into their heads to pester me. I must eat. Must, Must, Must. I have heard that word too often! I can't take any more of this pressure! I have had enough! I won't eat. I have eaten too much already lately. So much that the sight of all this food makes me feel sick.

Lætitia recommends the fish. According to her it is one of the few more-or-less edible dishes. She finishes everything in her containers with all the frenzy of someone who knows their life depends on it. She seems quite cheerful, despite the hurtful remarks Kevin manages to direct at everyone in the group. Zoë is quiet. She eats her meal in silence. She makes me think of a big, jolly teddy bear. And yet she has an almost apologetic air about her. She looks as if she has fallen down a hole and resigned herself to staying there. Houda takes no notice of anyone. She is permanently on the defensive, observing. Claire is looking for something to hold onto. She arrived the same day I did, during the afternoon. She seems completely disorientated. As for Fabien, he is apparently trying to break the human record for wolfing down food. It is enough to put off even someone who does have an appetite…

I hear the others talking. I watch and listen to them with the objectivity of a scientist presented with a complex problem. They are talking about weight. The discussion was triggered by my arrival. Charlotte thinks she is too fat and should go on a diet, but she lacks resolve and keeps putting it off. This frustrates her, and because she eats when she feels bad she continues to put on weight. I don't think she is all that fat.

In my eyes I am the only problem on earth because everyone else manages to live. I would like to be cured too. But it has to be other people who cure me. I can't fight any more. I can't rid myself of the frightening feeling of being an onlooker in my own life, of other people deciding for me. It makes my head spin. I feel as if I am trapped in a hideous body that no longer has any control over itself; it is enslaved to the will of others. This feeling has grown since I came into hospital. I really don't have any control over anything in here. No one even asked me whether I wanted to go on the walk, they simply didn't tell me. I count for nothing. I am worthless, ineffectual.

The only effect I have is the pain I cause others, which is why they stuck me in here. And now the doctors have to 'save' me so that the little package my parents left to be serviced can be returned to them in working order. Otherwise Package will be packed off to a long-stay hospital.

The meal is over. The trays are piled up, the cutlery cleared away and everyone goes back to their rooms. I don't feel like following the general movement. Going back to my room means being subjected to more of Houda's music, and I heard enough of that last night. I prefer to stay here. Unfortunately, the medical team objects to me not doing what the others do, and when the nursing staff see me sitting alone in the canteen having strayed from their nice, orderly flock, a whole group of them gather round and try to smooth-talk me into rejoining it; I mustn't forget how frail I am, etc.

# 11

2pm. It is still Tuesday. A day can be never-ending. Especially when you spend it on your own contemplating the gloom. I have given up looking outside for a brighter patch of cloud that would show me where the sun is. I don't know when it will finally deign to go down. Hurry, sun! Hide! So that I can escape this pointless life into the oblivion of sleep, even though I don't dream any more. Sleep: that world without happiness and joy reflecting how little there is in reality!

'Hope.' There's a vague word. What are you supposed to be hoping for when you hope? I would like to be able to hope but I can't. It's not my fault. I just can't. All I know is it's impossible. I need help. But not from doctors. I have seen too many of them. They don't help me, they just examine me. I need a guide, someone to show me the way back to life. Because at the present moment no one could argue that I am alive, what with my morbid reflections and my skeletal appearance. People are scared of me. They avoid me with a nervous smile or a pained expression before continuing on their way.

There is no point in asking people I know for help. They can't help me. They don't understand me. They never even noticed how bad I felt, how unhealthy my relationship to life had become. Did they even realise I existed? In any case they wouldn't have time to help me. They have their own worries and concerns... And I prefer not to bother them. I have bothered enough people already. I feel I am cheating someone else out of a place here; there are so many cases waiting to be admitted. Then again, I am sparing my family the pain of watching me waste away. And they don't have to worry about me because I am in here, where there's nothing to do except cry.

I am going to ask a priest to come and see me. He will tell me what to do. I must find out how to arrange it. But for now, I am still not allowed any visitors – the 48 hours are not up yet.

# 12

4.30pm. Tea-time. Everyone rushes to the canteen and grabs a chair at one of the two round tables. I drag myself there without protesting and sit down. I accept my snack, which I hand discreetly to Fabien who is eternally grateful. Karim brings us the hot chocolate he has prepared with a machine using powdered milk. The cakes are quickly demolished; ditto the fruit juice and hot chocolate. The baby birds cry out for more. It's cold on the ward and they need their energy!

There is a discussion with the nurses. Are they allowed seconds? The baby birds argue their case and win. Then they talk about themselves a little, about their lives, how they hope to leave here soon. I listen. Lætitia is doing most of the talking today. She knows she will be leaving soon. She tells us about the home she is in. It is strange to hear the word 'home' being used to refer to something that isn't a home in the way I know it. I feel very different from the others, who find me perfectly normal. I realise how lucky I was being born into a close-knit family: Fabien's brother is seriously ill, Claire's mother has never really looked after her properly, and the others are in homes. I feel a bit lost when I am with them, even though they talk openly in front of me and don't leave me out.

# 13

Back in my room. I see from the timetable that tomorrow I will undergo a 'therapeutic activity'. I am not exactly thrilled, but I am keen to know what it might mean. Also, by the time I am there another day and a half of my life will be over.

I continue to do nothing – there is nothing to do. And my little voice has all the space it needs to make itself heard in this emptiness; I am sucked into the void of my thoughts. I brood over my life, my unhappiness, this neglect – I cannot escape, I keep coming back to myself. I only know that I am impure, unworthy to live like other people. And yet they do not notice my impurity or their own. They are naïve. I am too lucid. And I am not a good person, I even make others suffer: it devastates my parents to see me so unhappy, and the others feel sorry for them. I am a burden on all of them. I am despicable.

I cry. I hate myself. I hate this body I can't control. My clothes hang off me, and I am not remotely pretty. I look like a homeless person. Where is that pallid beauty I aspire? All I have are big, dark furrows round my weary-looking eyes, and my jaw and cheekbones jut out. I don't like my new haircut either. I used to have hair down to my waist. Now it is shoulder-length, and it doesn't suit me. But I didn't like it before either so I changed it. They say hair saps your energy and I thought I would look good with a bob. So I happily sacrificed my riches. And now I look even uglier. But it's too late. It will take ages to grow back!

I don't expect to be here by then. The best way to die would be to evaporate, if that was possible. I would be like a spirit, completely detached from my body, whose atoms would no longer exist. Blown away, scattered to the four winds! Free! I would see everything but no one would see me, or touch me. I would feed off images and beauty, sea spray and storms, gusts and gentle breezes. Listen to the sounds of nature and birds singing, dissolve into the sunset, gather pollen with the bees, become drunk on the dance of life and the discovery of endless fresh beauties.

But soon I would see how deluded I had been. I would hear the cars, the factories and bombs, breathe in the carbon monoxide and insecticides, drink in the council blocks, shanty towns and concrete and be killed off by epidemics, dictators and people who only think about making money.

Sobs.

I look at my body – people always centre on themselves when they are unhappy. My legs are too fat. I haven't lost enough weight yet to enjoy complete freedom of movement – impossible with so much flesh. I make circles in the air with my legs: I already enjoy their supple, fluid movement in the air. Yet they feel so heavy! Exhausted, I let them flop onto the bed. I try again. The more tiring it is the more calories I will burn.

I long to be like gossamer floating on the wind. I must get rid of this weight, this flesh. I beat the air with my legs using rhythmic, gymnastic movements. At the same time I realise that if I achieve my ideal of true thinness, I won't have the strength to be happy or to live because I will have almost no flesh left. And yet I cannot live unless I am pure and perfect. What if I am perfect – dying even – because I am prepared to go all the way to fulfil my dream? Will people not pay attention to me then? Will they not admire my courage in renouncing everything to satisfy the strict demands of my ideal? And above all will they not love me because I am perfect, maybe, if indeed I am perfect in my semi-evaporated state?

In fact, I am waiting to be noticed, not cured. To be accepted for what I am and not what others would like me to be. I tried too hard to live up to other people's ideals. Now I am collapsing under the weight of my own. But in fact I am freer because I am the one doing the imposing – and the pain has almost become a pleasure.

Do you really expect me to agree with you when you say, 'How thin you are! You should eat more! You'd be much prettier!' With your pained expressions, your clumsy words, your attempts not to hurt my feelings...

Never any spontaneity! Never any honesty! Why can't you simply tell me I am beautiful, not 'to make her feel better, it'll do her good'? And if you don't think so then look away! Stop trying to engrave this image of the living dead in your memory. I'm not a museum exhibit. And above all I don't listen to other people! When you pester me with your well-meaning 'sensible' words you close off my ears to the outside – I have already sealed them on the inside.

Sobs.

My legs drop abruptly to the bed. I turn over, grabbing my pillow in a gesture of despair, ashamed at being too weak to withstand the world. I press my head into its horrid, bulky mass, crushing my face against it, and in my

deep, weary rage I hold my breath until I feel I am
suffocating; then I let everything out, bursting into floods
of tears and clutching the lumpy pillow like a doll, to
comfort myself. I rest my head on it, the tears slowly
running down my cheeks. I calm down. I accept that I am
alone.

# 14

6.30pm. Dinner-time. The usual farce. I don't eat
anything.

How can I when I feel as though I have just been on a
huge binge? That vile smell makes me almost want to be
sick.

The others glance up at me occasionally. Suddenly
Claire says gently, 'You need to eat, you know!' I shake my
head and give an almost inaudible sound. Thank you for
caring! Finally, someone who wants me to get well who
isn't a doctor, parent or adult – and who doesn't insist
when I say no.

I leave the table and go straight to bed. This time the
nurses have told Houda not to play her music because I
had no sleep last night.

I sleep like a log.

# 15

Wednesday morning 8am. I am woken by the drab light flooding the room as the shutters are opened, and by Karim's booming voice saying good morning.

I know they will force me to go to breakfast, so I go of my own accord. To avoid problems. At least I slept better last night.

There is a surprise waiting for me in the main area of the canteen. A strange ritual is in progress. I move closer. A weighing session! And there's one every morning!

I won't. I won't, I won't, I won't! I repeat to myself between clenched teeth. I don't want the others to see. Why can't they leave me alone!

Claire steps off the scales. She thinks she is too fat and says she is going on a diet. I climb on – slightly curious to know how much I weigh all the same.

40.8 kilos. The nurses aren't happy, 'That's not very much,' and of course, 'You must eat.' I feel rather proud because I have lost more weight since Friday. But I still have a long way to go!

The nurses demand an explanation, as if they didn't know why I am 'thin'! I play the game, replying innocently that I had no idea I weighed so little, and that five days ago I weighed 43 kilos. They don't seem very pleased – or convinced!

I see no point in this conversation so I stop reacting to

their scolding. It works and they finally shut up. I wait for my fellow teenagers to be weighed and then it is time for breakfast.

The others are shocked. You only weigh 40 kilos, they are thinking as they look me up and down, comparing my height with my weight. Then the usual chat resumes. I am beginning to get used to it: 'I am fed up with being in hospital.' 'I want to get out of here.' 'I wish I had some real chocolate.' 'Why've I got this crap bread instead of cereal like you?' 'The food here's total rubbish.' 'Where are you from?'

# 16

Houda bursts into the room and looks annoyed to find me in here, as if I were taking up all the space. I don't like still being a burden – on her now – and yet I feel almost defiant, as if she were being unfair, almost as if I had a right to have rights, a right to exist! But I don't! I only have my duty to my ideals! And I am upset simply because she doesn't live up to them.

She puts her music on again. A nurse comes and tells her to turn the volume down. She asks whether we are getting on all right. I resign myself to saying yes to avoid trouble, but Houda doesn't see it that way. She's had enough of me. She complains that I don't like her music, that I'm never out of the room and that I go to bed too early. She is upset and accuses me of being sneaky and touching her stuff. I start sobbing. They force me to reveal the awful truth: Houda's music does bother me, in fact I hate it. I break down and cry, ashamed at having confessed, and caused a row, and made a spectacle of myself. I can't get used to her either and I can't go on like this! Houda watches me. She has no sympathy for this snowflake melting before her eyes. She looks pleased with herself.

The nurse discusses it with the other staff, and they decide to put me in a room at the far end of the ward, next to the showers and toilets. Lætitia is in there, but she is leaving sometime today so I will be on my own.

I take all my things out of the cupboard and put them on the bed, which they wheel along to my new room. I let them do all the work – robbing me of the effort I could have made to burn a few more calories. I wore myself out getting worked up.

# 17

In reality, I have never been strong. I think I have always been weak. I never had to fight for anything. I did well at school, and in my other activities, because I was bright. If I hadn't been, I might have been forced to struggle, which would have allowed me to be stronger. As it is I am slowly letting go. I am tired of making efforts that lead nowhere.

Maybe you think life is easier if you are bright? I can assure you it is not. Especially when being bright means being 'able'. In fact, if you need problems in your life, then be 'able' – or 'gifted' if you prefer, even though I hate that word. It all started at secondary school. Or rather when I was conceived, since you don't become 'able' overnight: it is like a genetic disease you are born with, and stuck with, for the rest of your life. Don't worry, I am not planning to tell you my whole life story from day one. For a start I can't remember that far back, and not all of it is interesting.

In secondary school I was also top of my class, for a change! And believe me it isn't any fun. I'd already spent the whole of primary school trying to get used to being the 'teacher's pet'. Being the 'lucky' one who held the teacher's hand when we walked in a crocodile instead of a classmate's like everyone else; showing off my exercise books to the rest of the class and being applauded at the teacher's request by pupils who couldn't care less about my beautiful handwriting, and finally, being hated by all those pupils because of these 'privileges' which I would have gladly given up! Yes, I did well at school but I never asked for all that.

So I had had enough. School is no fun when you can guess what the teacher is going to say before he opens his mouth. I decided to do something about it. I asked to skip a year. Yes, me, all by myself! 'What? Skip a year! And in secondary school! You'll be behind! You'll never catch up! What about your friends?' But I hated being bored in class. It was driving me mad. I was prepared to try anything to get out of that situation. And it wasn't my parents being pushy that made me ask. It really was my decision. In any case, I didn't have many friends. All I risked was making some new ones.

My parents and I managed to convince the headmaster, and the following term I went straight into the third year at secondary school. It really was a great year, and I made a lot of friends. I was no longer top of the class and I enjoyed lessons because learning had become a challenge. I wanted to prove that they had been right to believe in me, and I needed to prove to myself I could do it.

Now I don't even know what school is for any more. To open people's minds? Yes, but to what? To the knowledge of their inevitable decay? To all the horrors man perpetrates? To their feelings, as futile as their appearance? What is the use of studying if you cannot take your knowledge with you when you die? To make money and friends? But why, if we have to leave everything behind on earth?

There it goes again, my little voice with its endless, exhausting thoughts. Why can't they make them stop? I can't bear it any more. I wish I could tear my brain out. These thoughts are evil; they multiply, destroying everything in their path, gnawing away steadily, faster and faster, at the furthest corners of my imagination, covering my thoughts and memories in a grey veil, gloomy and sad like a rainy day.

I feel completely detached. As if I were looking at someone else's thoughts and feelings from the outside. What is the point of having feelings anyway, if they only make you suffer?

# 18

My new room is bigger and green. Dingy, to be precise, as much because of the colour as the atmosphere. Facing the door in the middle of the wall is a large window decorated with black iron bars. It looks onto a grey building that probably hasn't been repainted since it was first built – which clearly wasn't yesterday. If I go closer, I can see the rooftop with its assorted chimney stacks and aerials poking up at the sky like the gnarled fingers of a witch against an endless expanse of grey. The chimney stacks have an abandoned look about them, decaying and beyond repair, like me.

I have to put my things away, which doesn't take long, and then I lie down on the bed and start crying again. I spend my whole life breaking down. Houda is hateful, I am pathetic, and no one cares about me. Too bad. In any case I am worthless. I should just die. How sad! I would so like to have been happy, wouldn't I, little voice? Why couldn't I have been blind and insensitive like the others and gone on living as though everything were all right?

I am getting nowhere either: I am still just as fat, and I can't fight any more. I am fed up with the cowardly looks people give me and the forced pity on their faces. I don't know whether doctors have to swear an oath that says, 'I promise I shall always look blankly at patients whoever they may be.' If not it must come with the job.

But my main cause of despair is still me: this body and soul called Mathilde with no distinction made between the two. I would so love to exist truly, to be valued by somebody. Why can't I be like other people and have friends? Why does no one ever call me? It isn't fair. It must be my fault.

I am not energetic enough, I am too frail. No! It isn't because of my weight: I know that what counts is a girl's body not her eyes. This is why I owe it to myself to be perfect, so that I will be attractive and people will notice me.

I have already tried to be funny, kind, sweet, understanding and whatever else I could be. But the only compliments it got me were: she's a 'dependable' or an 'intelligent' girl. Basically, a brainbox. It is not my fault! I didn't ask to have a mind like a salad spinner going round in circles and making everyone dizzy, and so full of leaves that they get shredded and fly all over the place when the lid is taken off, making it impossible to find out what went wrong and fix it!

# 19

I shower, return to my room, remove the wisps of lank hair hanging like rats' tails from my hairbrush and add a few new strands.

And now to more serious matters. I mustn't stop at 40 kilos. I must continue making headway. I am going to exercise, to lose more weight – I should have some muscles left after 10 years of ballet classes, even if I have lost 13 kilos!

To work! I lean on the radiator in front of the window (it's more fun) and begin meticulously practising my pliés, making sure I am in the proper position and above all trying to tense as many muscles as possible. It's tiring but I persist. It's good to have an aim in life! And I have nothing else to do. I move on to my 'attitudes'. I lift my leg in the air with my knee bent, facing upwards. Forward, side, back, next leg! Then my arabesques.

Now that I feel really tired, I lie down on the bed and repeat the exercises I was doing last night: lifting and lowering my legs alternately, pedalling in the air, tensing all my muscles and opening my legs in a scissor position... I am stiff all over from the effort. You have to suffer to be beautiful: sad but true.

Suddenly there is a knock at the door. I let my legs fall to the bed like dead weights. No one must know. It is my secret. Otherwise I will be in trouble. I love exercising, especially when it is really strenuous, I mean when I do it on an (almost) empty stomach.

It is Catherine the nurse again. I am intrigued. She is pushing a visibly heavy trolley, covered in a myriad of wires connected to various clips and boxes; I guess that this must be the electrocardiogram they have been promising me. I am impatient to see how it works, and what the result will be. If only my heart would slow down; it is beating so fast after all the exercise I have been doing. I am going to get a good reading but it will be the wrong one! I wish my heart could beat very slowly, as if I were terribly weak, which I am obviously not yet or I wouldn't be capable of all this physical effort.

Catherine begins untangling the wires and explains that she is going to tape some patches to my body and connect them via the wires – if she can unravel them – to the box that will measure my ECG. She tapes on the patches (legs, chest, lower body) then connects them to the transmitter wires. I have to hold my breath, relax and keep still. I do as I am told.

The first attempt fails. There's a problem, I don't know why but there is. The second attempt also fails. I am really beginning to enjoy this. And it helps pass the time, the same as meals but less unpleasant and no one is pressurising me to eat. Third attempt. Not great apparently but it'll do. What a shame, I would have liked another go. Too bad, at last I will be alone again, away from this stranger's eyes staring at me.

Catherine peels off the bits of tape. 'There we are, and you get a free waxing into the bargain,' she quips, although this is completely untrue as the tape comes off without tearing any hairs out. She was just trying to make conversation. She is right, I am not exactly talkative.

Before going out she announces that Dr Crapaud has decided to put me on anti-depressants (it was to be expected!), and that I will need to undergo some tests to determine the proper dosage. This casts a slight chill over me, especially coming just after the little game with the ECG. I have no desire to be in the grip of a drug that is capable of making me think differently. I would rather be put on a drip. It feels as if they are prescribing a lobotomy: they are going to take away my thoughts, take *me* away. I feel bad enough about being in my body already without them having to eradicate my thoughts too. What is this? Am I really that far gone? Can they find no other way of curing me except through drugs?

I deeply regret having come into hospital. More than ever I feel they want to get rid of me. I tell myself I shall no longer be free. I want to continue being me, I don't want to be on some drug that will make me think properly and take away my freedom. Besides, if it is the anti-depressant making me happy then I am not really cured – I mean, if I were really cured I wouldn't need drugs to be happy. I don't want to be dependent, I want to be free! I don't mind so much being locked up in hospital, but the thought of them imprisoning my imagination is unbearable. Then again, I knew this was likely to happen; it was one of the risks I took by coming here. And it is a sort of challenge, something new. I am so unresponsive and they are so desperate for a solution that they have to put me on an anti-depressant, so it is also a victory, or rather another phase.

All the same I want my thoughts to be free. Dr Crapaud hasn't seen me again since our first appointment before I was admitted. On what authority has she based her decision? I know she isn't the slightest bit interested in me.

# 20

The day goes by with its round of cleaning, menus, mealtimes, silences, loneliness and futile thoughts I am unable to stop. In the evening, just before dinner, I take my anti-depressant for the first time; it's an orange-coloured syrup the nurses dilute before giving to me. It tastes sweet but not nice. It makes no difference to me. I keep it down, as if I thought it could offer me the hope I need, though without much conviction. Maybe I am just curious.

At 5pm I had my first visitor. Mum had apparently been waiting anxiously to see what sort of state she would find me in. She always worries about everything. I was in my room. I knew she would come as soon as I was allowed visitors, and that she missed me terribly. She didn't say this but I knew. I could see she was on edge, in a permanent state of nerves. It was silly of her. She was wearing herself out for no reason: I wasn't worried about leaving here, or living, so why should she be? In the name of supposedly instinctive motherly love? It's not something I can relate to. I shall never be a good mother. In fact, I shall never be a mother.

Mum's presence made me feel guilty. It was my fault she was anxious. I was to blame and I felt like a burden, which I hated, and I wished it would stop and that I could disappear. When I saw her, I felt so paralysed by the cold in the room and my own inner coldness that I didn't want her to hug me, but I let her, as though I no longer belonged to myself, as though my body and mind were no longer connected.

I sensed in her smile and in her embrace her desire to surround me with love, her need to comfort and protect me with her warmth. My body yielded but my mind was free. I couldn't let go – above all I had to stay in control.

I admit I was happy to see her though. No, not happy! Let's say pleased. She was the only person who really knew me. She would listen. Yet I chose my words carefully, changing the subject, concealing the painful thorn in my side. I didn't want her to suffer. I intended to be alone in my martyrdom to my ideals that were higher than those of the rest of mankind. And in any case she wouldn't have understood, she would have argued with me and her visit would have become a bore.

I told her about hospital life. Though to be honest there wasn't much to tell: the staff, the buildings, all of them cold. I told her how bad I felt, crying in my room all day surrounded by the other lonely teenagers. Of course we were all suffering too much to be of much help to one another, but I was the only one who kept my distance.

I told her about the photography workshop that afternoon. They sat us down on some exercise mats in a room opposite the ward, next to Dr Crapaud's office, then spread out some photos and pictures in plastic sleeves on the floor and asked us each to choose one and talk about it. I can't remember what I chose – landscapes, I think. Or faces. Some distant thing.

Then I told her about Lætitia leaving. At the time, shut away in my own world, I hadn't really thought about it, but later on that light at the end of the tunnel would prove decisive for me.

Mum asked whether I needed anything. I said I wanted some tissues and my bottle of scented face oil. And I suggested she bring me some clean clothes and take away my dirty ones. I also told her I was cold and wanted a sleeping bag.

And then it was time to say goodbye. We asked one of the nurses whether it was possible for me to see my local priest. No. I could see the hospital priest but I wasn't allowed visits from non-family members... So I would see the hospital priest.

# 21

Thursday. There is no therapeutic activity today because all the medical staff are in the fortnightly meeting. Only the auxiliary nurses, like Karim, are here to look after us.

I hate this place this morning. I really have to leave. I can't stand being controlled like a puppet any more, and I don't want to be on anti-depressants. I want to get better on my own. I know I am right. Even if this drug could help me I prefer to go it alone. And I would so like to be happy at last! Other people are, so why can't I be? I decide at breakfast to drink my orange juice and my mug of chocolate. I give the rest to the vultures at the table.

Thursday is sheet-changing day. We busily strip off our beds, separating the sheets and pillowcases from the blankets, and remake them with clean linen. Then we lie down again.

I spend the rest of the morning re-reading the hospital rules. There is a timetable of 'therapeutic activities'. Monday: theatre; Tuesday: outing; Wednesday: photo and story workshop alternately; Thursday: nothing; Friday and Saturday: arts and crafts. On Sundays there are outings, and some people go home, but never on the first Sunday.

We are gathered in the canteen waiting for lunch when the medical staff emerge from the nurses' station. Dr Crapaud goes over to Houda and tells her she is being discharged. Houda, overjoyed, races to her room to pack

62

her bags; she will be leaving in the late afternoon. I am amazed by the way they discharge a patient. (I had some intense sessions with Houda and I feel far more affected by her leaving than I did when Lætitia left.) The decision was taken so quickly. Indeed, Lætitia's departure and then Houda's raise my own hopes of leaving here quickly.

I decide to eat some lunch as well. I find it difficult, but I know it's the price I must pay if I want to be discharged. They have made this much clear to me! As I leave the table it occurs to me how truly awful the food here is; if they are expecting to give anorexics their appetites back with this type of concoction they must think they'll swallow anything.

I go back to my room; a lot of us have a siesta after lunch. I feel strangely torn. I have a sense of triumph, like the victorious knight who has slain the dragon and is about to present its head to the hideous hag Dr Crapaud in order to win the hand of Lady Liberty. And at the same time I feel I have given up just when I was about to achieve my goal. Yes, I gave in! It took me two months to reach this state of total starvation, and from one day to the next I start eating again!

Also, I am in hospital, which is surely a sign of having achieved something through my efforts: I have starved myself enough for people to notice. Should I give it all up now?

It must be three weeks including half-term since I last went to school, and yet Mum hasn't mentioned anyone asking about me. I feel I don't count for anything. When you are unhappy people don't want to know. Almost no one except my family cares about me, or should I say is lumbered with me.

Stop, little voice! You're hurting me!

Objectively speaking, I managed to swallow my pride and eat, with the sole aim of escaping from the hospital, instead of from the world as I had wanted to up until then. Lætitia's life-affirming smile when she was about to leave convinced me happiness exists and I must try to find it – even if no one else cares and I am only doing it for myself. Staying in hospital won't make me happy and my family are suffering because they are paying for me to be here.

And besides, isn't happiness one of my ideals? Yes. Together with nature, beauty, truth, love, purity and dignity. But if these values, which some people think are old-fashioned or useless, aren't instinctive in me, I won't make them any more so by running away; on the contrary, I must be an example. It's a shame I have to eat in order to leave! But this is what I want, so I am going to do it!

My stomach feels funny, not very nice, but I know it's because I haven't eaten for so long. Suddenly, I am afraid of putting on weight and I do my exercises again, the same as yesterday.

While I am doing the movements I follow a train of thought: destination nowhere. Mum said she would bring me some books as well as clothes. This won't be until Friday because the nurse thinks it is better for me not to see her every day. It doesn't bother me. I am the solitary type and I have never missed anyone.

I am hoping I will tone up a bit, but in fact I am too weak to be able to do the movements properly, tensing my muscles. I tell myself that eating will give me more energy, but I have to be rigorous about doing my exercises so that I develop muscles and not fat.

# 22

I will spare you the details of tea-time. Suffice it to say that since I have already eaten I force myself on principle to drink some fruit juice. When you decide to do something, especially if it requires a huge effort, it is best to start straight away.

After tea, Claire suggests we play a board game. We choose Monopoly, as it is the only game which doesn't have half its pieces missing. We sit in the canteen huddled round one of the tables. After a while everyone has had enough – everyone being Claire, Houda, Fabien, Zoë, Kevin, and me – and we decide to talk instead, but in our rooms so Karim won't be breathing down our necks.

We all tell our story. Mine is pathetic. They have real reasons for being unhappy: orphaned, parents divorced, too much family pressure, not enough love, a little brother who is dying, drugs! My depression seems selfish by comparison. Everyone has revealed something about themselves, and I feel obliged to as well. But I don't know what to say. My problems seem so trivial compared to theirs. I tell them I am the eldest child of a large family, and that I wore myself out by taking on too much responsibility, and that my dad is away a lot because he is in the navy. I say all this to hide the fact that my unhappiness isn't caused by external factors. I know that none of this is making me ill. The problem is me. Me and my tormented thoughts. But there's no way of stopping thinking, and anyway I wouldn't want to.

Then something incredible happens that amazes and astonishes me: they respond as one and comfort me! They say nice things to me and tell me they also feel cowardly and despicable moaning while other children are dying of hunger, and they don't understand why they are in this state when relatively speaking they could be leading perfectly normal lives like everyone else, and they know they are doing no one any good being like this. Yes, they respect me, and what makes me different, and they hope I get better because they identify with me, they know what suffering is. There are no gratuitous words or gestures; only Charlotte who is sitting next to me gently places her hand on my shoulder. There is no place for shame or judgement as each listens to the feelings and experiences of the others and talks about their own. This strengthens us. We are a group of walking wounded huddled together on a couple of hospital beds.

We each confide our fears, our frustration with life and our need for friendship, our desire to get out of this hospital, this hell, and our hopes of being happy. We aren't friends, but a group of people who have been brought together and are helping one another.

It is a beautiful moment and it restores my faith in life. Afterwards, Houda takes her things into the hall. We all feel sad. She was an important part of our group, even though not everyone always got along with her. She at least deserves credit for having livened up this deadly place and her departure will affect us far more than Lætitia's did. We are happy for her and there are no hard feelings because we all have problems and understand her rebellion. But we are torn between the vague hope of getting out of here one day and the sad fact of our despair at being left behind. One by one the others go back to their rooms, but I am unable to tear myself away from this girl who draws me irresistibly to the outside world.

I am sitting down. Houda sits next to me. It is the first time we have really talked. The only thing she ever told me was that she lived in a home. She doesn't apologise. Neither do I. It doesn't matter now: at moments like these there is no place for petty past differences. She simply makes me promise I will eat and be happy and I tell her I hope she has a good life.

Our words are shallow yet they possess the depth of language that links two people who have nothing in common. I remember this moment (I want to describe it) as if it were a still photograph, a faded image of a moment in time, like a fond memory. It is the image I wish to keep of her. She did have a heart, and she showed it to me. I think that of everyone on the ward I had the hardest time with her. Her music, her arrogance and her aggressive language were not easy for any of us to live with, but I was too different from her to be able to adjust to her in the way the others did. And yet I was the only one she opened up to.

That evening I ate and took my medication without protesting. Our table was quiet, as if the secrets we had each confided about our suffering still echoed in the silence, and the usual round of complaints had no place.

# 23

Friday. I have my first real meeting with a member of the medical team since I arrived: the psychologist. I see her coming from a distance, dressed in black leather against the white walls, gliding 10 centimetres above the ground, her platinum blonde hair and the indelible impression of her bright-red lipstick floating behind her.

I am watching from her office opposite the ward, next to Dr Crapaud's office.

'Good morning. Sit down. What's your name?'

'Mathilde.'

'Oh! That's a pretty name! What does it mean?'

Stunned, I tell her that 'Mathilde' means 'mighty in battle'. I am expecting the usual response, 'That's not very ladylike,' or something, but to my amazement she comes back with, 'Hm! And what is your particular battle?' in a disconcertingly serious voice.

I am completely thrown. I have no idea how to answer this one. Literally or metaphorically? I choose the latter, to prove to her I am not mad and she must let me out of this prison immediately.

I launch into a little speech about how as a good Catholic I want to practise the Church's teachings by being kind and helping others, spreading the word of Jesus to anyone who wants to listen and generally being a model of harmony!

'Is this why you have stopped eating and are destroying yourself?'

Ouch! She is right, there is a slight contradiction. I change the subject, explaining to her my ideal of purity and self-denial: I want to be thin in order to conform to the current dictates of fashion, to be noticed and loved. I don't want to have cellulite! I am trying through self-denial and my detachment from my body to achieve a kind of purity, to distance myself from other human beings whose despicable behaviour sickens me.

'And how did you reach this point?'

69

# 24

I tell the psychologist about my life. I feel as if I am talking to myself. She takes notes on a big pad of paper and tries to form a picture of my family, my brothers and sisters, my problems, etc.

I am the eldest of six: four girls and two boys. Dad is in the navy and Mum is a housewife: I couldn't see her coping with a job as well, given the constant hubbub there is in our house. The three youngest are the worst offenders: Marc is forever provoking Maguelone while the little one thinks up new ways of being a nuisance. Maxime and Marion, aged 12 and 11, are weekly boarders, only coming home at weekends to monopolise our parents' attention. Meanwhile the three youngest demand their share of cuddles and throw tantrums because our parents are busy with the two bigger children.

The weekends are particularly difficult and stressful. Maxime and Marion arrive at 10pm on Friday and leave again at 3pm on Sunday. Saturday is taken up with shopping, and on Sunday morning we all go to Mass. So there is very little time to relax, or rather for them to relax and be made a fuss of by my parents because they are so sad to be leaving them for another week. My role in all this is to calm down Marc, Maguelone and Marguerite at the weekends, and to put up with the background noise of their shouting all week while I try to concentrate on my homework.

I sympathise with the little ones though. It is understandable they feel they aren't getting enough attention: during the week our parents are too busy for cuddles, and when the long-awaited weekend arrives the older children come and jump the queue. We all end up tired and irritable, and Maxime and Marion hardly help matters by moaning about how hard their lives are as boarders…

Maxime's and Marion's school is in Aubenas, in the Ardèche region. The round trip by train takes 10 hours, so they aren't exactly fresh for their lessons on Monday mornings. Why this absurd situation when right across the road there's a school that caters for pupils from nursery school right up to the end of secondary school? Well… it's because they are also 'gifted'. Unfortunately, the headmaster who had agreed to me skipping a year wasn't as flexible when it came to my brother and sister: this was the proof my parents were pushy! Also Maxime's and Marion's marks weren't as good as mine; school felt like a waste of time because they weren't fulfilling their potential, and they soon 'switched off'. They had to 'flunk out' before they were allowed to change schools. It was essential for them to skip a year in order to be re-motivated.

But it was already autumn half-term, and the only school prepared to bend the rules and accommodate them was 350 kilometres away from where we lived, in Aubenas. They ran a special programme for gifted children which allowed them to advance more quickly through secondary school. Marion started there in November, skipping two years thanks to their system, and Maxime followed her in January, skipping one year. And so brother and sister ended up in the same class. This would lead to other problems.

Meanwhile I continued alone at the school across the road with my younger brother and two sisters. Despite Marc, Maguelone and Marguerite's non-stop activity the evenings at home dragged, and the weekends weren't long enough, and were no picnic.

I had been taking ballet classes outside school since the age of four. It seems I was good at that too: I started dancing on points when I was seven and a half, and by the time I was 11, I was in a class with 16-year-olds. I was the 'baby' as far as they were concerned, although I didn't consider myself a baby at all; I didn't think talking about clothes between exercises was a sign of being grown up. The main difference between us, apart from our size, was that I needed to be constantly moving. While they discussed music or ballet steps with the teacher, a very sweet lady who was genuinely fond of me, I amused myself by sliding around on the parquet floor. The other girls were always criticising me and I had to sit still and be quiet because I was too young to be helping with the choreography. I loved dancing and I miss it now, but I felt terribly lonely during the classes.

I was also in the girl guides. Being a guide meant a lot to me. I could hardly wait to become patrol leader, to organise games and excursions, to share my love of nature with the girls in my patrol and teach them how to set up camp. I aimed to encourage a spirit of friendship and goodwill in my patrol. Last June I had to give it up. I was too run down because of that stupid glandular fever to take part in the summer camp. It was a huge disappointment to me. It was the best patrol I had ever been in. I couldn't go back this year, I was too weak.

I also tell the psychologist how much I like reading,

writing, singing and above all making things with my hands. Though unfortunately we don't have any materials for this at home, and in fact when I was small Mum never encouraged me to do painting and modelling. I suppose it was because she didn't like all the cleaning up afterwards. Nowadays it is difficult to do anything without my younger brothers and sisters getting in the way. When I am alone in my room, I draw or write poems or songs...

Then my friends left. I went back to school and studied until I was too exhausted and I stopped. Like with the ballet classes. I began my quest for purity, truth and goodness. I ate next to nothing. I took a bad fall and I'm not right in the head. And now I am waiting for someone to help me. But no one seems to understand this, and I must keep struggling and thinking. Alone. End of life story.

I leave the psychologist feeling even more confused. How can she help me? I feel as if I have just given a lecture on my family history and I know my subject well! I have been over the situation enough times in my head, twisting the knife endlessly in the wound.

And she never once stopped me to help me focus on some painful aspect I might not have seen or wanted to see on my own. She only interrupted me to ask for more details about my everyday life.

# 25

The psychologist walks me back to the canteen where the others are already having lunch. I find it slightly unnerving the way they always look at me as if they were seeing me for the first time, but it doesn't upset me since nothing really matters. Seeing them eating, their startled eyes turned towards me, I feel pity, as if I were seeing baby birds tortured by children. And in their collective gaze there is an air of that surprise and relative indifference to the possible suffering still in store for them. It is very strange: at times we feel so close, like allies, beyond the nurses' reach, and yet as soon as we are apart it is almost as though we had never met, as though we had to start all over again. Maybe all that unites us is our suffering and our shared relationship to the nurses.

On the other hand when they look at me I feel I exist. They are seeing me. It doesn't matter whether they are wondering how my meeting with the psychologist went or just watching me as they would a passing cloud. The main thing is their eyes are fixed on me; even if they do have that surprised look as though they had never seen me before, I am the one they are looking at.

I sit down and pick at my food.

# 26

The arts and crafts activity takes place in the mornings. I feel slightly frustrated not to have been yet. Painting, singing, writing and dancing are the only ways I have of relaxing and expressing myself. Ever since I was little I have had a need for these things. Since I caught glandular fever they have all stopped. The weight of fatigue paralysing my limbs trapped all my creative energy inside me.

People who have difficulty expressing or communicating their feelings sometimes compare themselves to a pressure cooker. I am more like a sponge. I love to soak up the beauty of the world and spray my feelings over everything around me. But the sponge has lost its strength, the energy that made my inner life, now stagnant, burst forth. The sponge went on soaking up until it drowned from having soaked up only painful things. And now instead of bursting forth, life seeps out in the form of exhausting tears. The sponge slowly empties, stops replenishing, dies a slow death. The tears trickle without soothing, burn like drops of white-hot metal, crystals of vanished happiness piercing the wounded child, destroying her, plunging her deeper into despair. Gradually the tears stop flowing. There is nothing left inside fine enough to seep through the tiny pores and the sponge dries up.

No, I didn't explode like a pressure cooker because I

had too many pent-up feelings inside. I would have needed strength in order to explode, and I haven't any. I don't even have that. And people would notice if I exploded. Yet everyone carries on as before. No one can see me because I have died inside. I imploded, and the implosion destroyed me; the outside world crushed me because I took it upon myself to try and alter it – and failed. This wounded me fatally, and I changed. I died inside.

I feel no bitterness when I think about this; it is part of who I am. Suffering strengthens us because we must triumph over it. I still believe my cause is worthy. The challenge is not to let it destroy me.

# 27

I feel like reading this afternoon. I don't know if I can wait until Mum brings me those books. Having nothing to do is so frustrating. Thinking hurts too much, and anyway, thinking while looking at these drab, dirty walls bathed in grey light is likely to make anyone go round in circles. In fact, there is nothing like it for tying your thoughts up in knots, the sort of knots that cut off the life supply to the brain.

I ask the nurses if there is a library at the hospital. One of them gives me the key to the cabinet in the canteen and tells me to write down my name, the date and the title of the book I borrow in a small pad.

What books did I read? All I remember is I went through them at a terrific speed. It is true I had nothing else to do except for my exercises, which took up very little time. There was one book of strange stories – by Mark Twain, I think – which I found absorbing. There were other books too, of course, but I have forgotten what they were. In fact, reading was no more important to me than my other activities. All I wanted was to get out of there. And I still hadn't seen Dr Crapaud! It was beyond me. This feeling of being left to die like in an old people's home.

It seems the Celts used to put sick people in a hut outside the village and take them soup every day. Whether they were cured or not was left in the lap of the gods. I sympathise with those people left to end their lives alone.

# 28

We were having tea when Manu arrived. He looked almost as lost as I did, but a lot unhappier, as if he were about to burst into tears. He went to unpack his things and came back later to join us.

'Why are you here?' someone blurts out, after he has told us his name.

He doesn't feel like talking. I think he is probably suffering from depression. He soon divides his time, like Fabien, Claire, Zoë and Kevin, between the smoking room, the TV and his bed – which is to say we don't see much of each other.

There is a big upheaval on the ward that evening because Kevin, who is delighted, is also leaving: the general feeling is one of relief as his explosive personality disturbed the 'peace' of the ward, which wasn't to the liking of the other inhabitants and had already caused a few rows.

The same evening small, feisty Fleur arrives. There is a look of determination and pain in her eyes and when she pierces you with her gaze you feel ashamed for daring to look at her because her suffering is so much greater than yours. She is like a proud stallion, a gypsy or an African chief, and I am unable to take my eyes off her because she fascinates me.

We are told another boy is arriving tomorrow morning,

another depressive. This ward seems to specialise in them. There are only five rooms, three doubles and two singles, and they will need to be allocated differently. I will be sharing with Fleur, which I am slightly dreading.

# 29

The same day, Friday. Mum comes to see me for the second time. She arrives half an hour late because of all the shopping she had to do for me. I am not annoyed with her. She has brought a sleeping bag, a personal CD player, my CDs and some clothes; she couldn't find much in my wardrobe, and appears to have cleaned out an entire clothes shop. I don't like the styles she has chosen and the colours are boring, but I am pleased: she has gone to a lot of trouble for me and I tell her how pretty everything is.

She has also bought me a hair clip and a hair stick; I used to like putting my hair up with a stick when it was long. Mum meant well, and to show my enthusiasm I try to fasten my hair with it, but it's no use – my hair is too short and it won't stay up. I think I look distinctly ugly with this new haircut, and now I can't manage to look remotely like my old self even with the aid of this favourite object.

Mum senses she has hurt me without meaning to, and assures me my hair will grow back. I think of the strands clogging my brush every morning or which I find on my clothes.

I look through the CDs she has brought me: The Cranberries, Norah Jones, Dido, Carla Bruni. It is good to have them, but at the same time I don't see the point. In fact, I never really listen to music. I prefer silence. Or singing songs I make up as I go along which flow out of me like spring water, purifying me. I don't really identify with the words and music of any singers.

I shall lend my CDs to the others; they are always asking me what my favourite music is. To be honest I don't know much about music. I only know rap and R&B from hearing it on their radios. I was brought up with older French singers like Joe Dassin or Alain Souchon.

From an early age the small amount of music I did listen to was classical. It was enough for me. I loved being transported by those sounds that gave me the freedom I needed to dream. I didn't even know who the composers were. It was the music I heard during ballet class, and which made me want to pirouette and fly through the air. I invented words for it and wrote and re-wrote them according to the mood I was in.

Just before she leaves Mum gives me the bottle of face oil I asked her for. The lavender scent still evokes the hospital for me, immersing me in sad memories.

To put her mind at rest Mum asks Brigitte the nurse whether I am allowed a sleeping bag. The answer is no. She takes the bulky bag away with her and I wave goodbye to my nights snuggled up in that familiar warmth. The nurses give me some blankets. They can't understand why I didn't ask for any before.

Antidepressant medication, then supper.

I am trying to fall asleep when Karim comes to fetch me around 9.30pm. According to him I spend too much time on my own and I sleep too much. I should go and join the others in the canteen where they are having a 'snack'.

I begin by refusing, then reluctantly give in and follow him there. There are cakes on the table, sponge cakes, and some other cakes in wrappers – the sort they always have in hospitals. Karim brings us a jug of hot chocolate. It smells good. I hate eating, but I love smells: the smell of bakeries and sweetshops, of beaches and pine trees. The smell of hospital...

I don't eat anything. I have already eaten today. I listen to the others talking. I love that feeling of being invisible and watching events unfolding before me, like being at the cinema. I don't speak, I am almost asleep.

At first my silence inhibits the others, but they are soon laughing and joking, enjoying themselves – like kids in the playground. I feel apart from them.

When this moment has passed, a split second in my memory, I head straight back to bed. There won't be any more 'snacks' for me. I am decidedly not cut out for life – not normal life, anyway. I make up my mind not to worry about what other people think. I will be me. I will live in order to prove that I don't need to give in to their way of doing things. I can be me.

# 30

Saturday morning. A lot of people are going home for the weekend. These days of 'rest' are when we are most left to our own devices. At breakfast, the joy on the faces of the people going away is distressing for those of us left behind. The ward goes quiet, deserted by its half-alive inhabitants who won't be here much longer (you are only allowed home for the weekend if you are on the road to recovery), and haunted by the ghosts of those who remain. Most of the medical staff are off duty too. The whole place is even emptier and bleaker than usual.

I press my face up against the window in the canteen that overlooks the car park. The sky is interminably grey, the trees in the park by the hospital chapel interminably black. A tall, dark building towering above the chapel appears in its imposing gloom to be trying to compete with our despair.

The car park is nearly empty. Everyone has gone. I gaze at the austere buildings and think of all the people dying in them. I feel that nothing has any meaning. Loneliness ought to be forbidden.

# 31

All the same, we are allowed to do arts and crafts this morning. One of the nurses, Catherine, brings a trolley laden with paints, paintbrushes, crayons, sticky tape, scissors, bits of papers and magazines.

It is November, and the idea is to make Christmas decorations for the ward. Fleur takes some tissue paper and makes a snow-scene based on a picture in a magazine. Manu draws something, I don't remember what. The others are away. I do what Catherine suggests and make a figure of Mary and Joseph out of wire and plaster. She looks lovely in the picture. I set to work.

We talk amongst ourselves. I discover that Fleur has already been in here once. But mostly it is the others who make me talk. Catherine is very sweet. She asks me questions about myself and my family and about arts and crafts, which she can see I enjoy. She says I have a flair for it. I don't know why. I don't think I am all that good at it. I just like looking, trying to see and under-stand what people are feeling so I can reproduce their expressions.

I chat away. It is very pleasant. Another nurse, Brigitte, arrives. It is as if a veil of intimacy has been created around the five of us. I love it when people take pleasure in slowly and painlessly lifting the curtain that divides them so that they can gradually get to know one another.

# 32

The boy they told us about arrived this morning. His name is Léon. As far as I can tell he just looks lost. Like the rest of us, he is in here because of depression.

Lunchtime.

I spend the afternoon reading.

After tea, I talk to Fleur. She is always doing acrobatics, aerial flips followed by the splits. She tells me she was a champion gymnast – this explains her small, muscular build. She talks a lot about horses too. She has put posters of them up in our room. Her dream is to become a riding teacher, and she already has her own horse. She also talks about her two suicide attempts.

I feel pathetic: Fleur has never known her father and she doesn't get on with her mother. She talks a lot about freedom. I have none of these problems and all I can do is cry.

# 33

They promise us that tomorrow we will do 'something' – go to the cinema or to McDonald's or somewhere. In the meantime I watch Karim and Fleur playing table-football. I am standing in order to burn more calories.

I want to start eating again, slowly, but I must exercise to build up my muscles. I don't want any fat on my body. This is why I no longer eat butter, oil or eggs: they disgust me. I am also careful to cut all the fat off my meat and not to eat too much starch. And I never touch sauces because they add calories to a meal.

It drives the others mad to see me standing all the time. It doesn't make me tired. Or maybe it does but I am so naturally exhausted these days anyway I don't even notice the slight difference this further effort makes.

I really am always tired. Looking back, I don't know how my legs carried me through that dark period of my life. When I was at my weakest they would give way and I would collapse, as if I had suddenly become paralysed. It was very peculiar. But at the time I was so wrapped up in my convictions and my ideals that in spite of my extreme fatigue I managed to keep going through sheer willpower. It was the same single-mindedness that allowed me to read.

I still have difficulty thinking, although since I made up my mind to live, that feeling of emptiness in my head is slowly going away. It terrifies me because it takes my soul away. I am no longer me. *Non cogito ergo non sum*. I have always thought a lot, and questioned things. The sum total of answers led me to conclude that my life is empty. Meaningless. The world outside is mad, selfish, without ideals or values, like that ball rolling randomly around the table.

I don't want this. My life needs some purpose. I am tired of hearing the words to all those empty songs because they don't bring any action. Action for me means sacrificing myself for my cause – for Goodness and Beauty. I have a vital need to give myself, to be an example to others. I don't expect people to follow my example, they have disappointed me too often for that, and I know they don't have the courage – they are too attached to their material comforts and possessions. No. I only hope that people will notice me, that my actions will make them think and, who knows, that they might even love me for who I am – though this seems so unbelievable I hardly dare put it into words.

I also have an unhealthy need for affection. I feel stifled at home. Smothered by the love of a mother who watches everything I do, as if she were afraid I might break in two, as if she were waiting to catch me in case I fall, as if she no longer trusted me. She is constantly telling me, 'You think you're right, but you twist everything. You only see the bad in things, and you end up hurting yourself.' And her endless insistence that I am wrong makes me stop listening to her or believing anything she says. I suppose she is still trying to protect me from reality, to convince me there is good in human beings, and between them. But I don't want some saccharine version of reality. I want reality, pure and simple, no half-measures. I want to face evil and fight it, not compromise. I want to be totally pure, so my purity shows on my face.

In spite of all her efforts, Mum doesn't give me any real affection. Simply because she doesn't accept me as I am. She needs me to behave 'properly' – i.e. not to question things and to live and be happy like everyone else, for my own good. I feel completely cut off from her. And anyway, how could I believe her? I am her daughter and she sees me through the distorting lens of a mother's love; I could be the ugliest daughter in the world and she would say I am the prettiest. But I don't want that. I prefer facing up to harsh reality than living in ignorance.

# 34

My period of self-sacrifice. The more desperately I tried to do all the little chores I thought would make life easier for my family (clearing the table, tidying the bathroom and kitchen, etc.) the less they noticed me. Instead of thanking me Mum would say, 'You'll wear yourself out, go and rest. I'll do that.' As for the others, they never even glanced up from the TV or computer or whatever game they were playing, they took everything I did for granted. I felt I didn't exist since I saw no reflection of my worth in any of their faces.

I tried to make myself pretty in the hope that people would notice me and like me, and I would have friends. This is also why I gradually reduced my calorie intake and was careful about what I ate. I invented a hundred reasons to run up and down the stairs every day, which wasn't too difficult as my bedroom was on the second floor. Yet for people around me, those for whom I was sacrificing myself, I felt I was slowly disappearing.

I worked hard on my assignments too. I wanted to be perfect on every level. I dreamed that through my purity I would become unattainable, above this world, and that those for whom I was prepared to lower myself – if only to win their love – would finally love me.

As time went by I became more and more lifeless. A simple remark would make me burst into tears at any moment. But instead of seeing this life draining from my eyes as a cry for help, people ran away. Out of embarrassment, or fear of suffering? Occasionally when this happened somebody would offer me a tissue and say, 'You'll get over it.' But that was all. Of course I would get over it. I'd be dead soon. Then I'd be over it.

As my life ebbed away I began to cry less. I had no tears left. In fact, I avoided drinking so I wouldn't be polluted by the act of going to the toilet. I had to remain pure at all times, especially since everyone else insisted on wallowing in their own dirt.

Occasionally I even stopped having thoughts altogether. My mind went blank. My physical self-denial had affected my brain, and sometimes I was only capable of mechanical, almost instinctive actions: standing, sitting or lying down, waiting for the time to pass; looking; answering an occasional question. It was like chasing white birds in the fog. I was searching blindly for the thoughts which eluded me. Thinking was impossible. Maybe that is what an animal is: someone who can't think. It wouldn't be so bad if you didn't already know what thinking is.

Drained and exhausted both physically and mentally, I was no longer in a condition to help other people. And so I decided that up until my imminent death I would avoid causing them any further problems, rather than trying to make them forget I was there, which they already had. For example: there was no need for them to lay my place at the table as I wasn't going to eat. I couldn't understand why this upset them, since it was my choice.

I wasn't happy at all. In fact, I suffered a lot. When I cried no tears came as I had nothing more to give. My skin and eyes were dried up and my heart was clammy and cold from lack of love. And yet I knew what I was doing. I knew I could expect nothing from the world and that I couldn't live with all its cowardliness, injustice and lies. I had tried to change things and influence others by changing myself, only to realise my struggle was in vain. People didn't want to be better themselves; they confirmed to me the horror of the world and the uselessness of my efforts. I refused to live like that, like them, and since I couldn't win my battle I preferred not to carry on being a burden to others by prolonging my futile struggle. I selfishly chose peace and suffered from loneliness and incomprehension.

I ended up in hospital almost by chance, as though catapulted there by some invisible force. I only agreed to go to please my parents; I told myself it would be less of a strain on them. It made no difference to me whether I was at home or in hospital. And maybe somewhere deep down I felt a tiny flicker of hope, which I didn't even dare put into words for fear of being disappointed in case it came to nothing.

I told myself God had given me life, and that I ought to be happy. But how? Why?

I told myself that I must try to eat and compensate by doing exercise. This way I would be both beautiful and healthy. I realised I was alone and I no longer expected any help from other people, though I accepted they were there.

# 35

The hospital was a strange place. Cold, silent, with the occasional sound of shouting or crying. There were teenagers from all over the region and from all different backgrounds. It was there I gained a deeper understanding of the reality of society: we were all affected. Society was harmful and destructive for us all.

But I also met teenagers who had a strong sense of identity, teenagers with dreams and hearts. They were rebelling against their parents, had problems at school, and suffered other hardships that are often talked about but whose impacts are unknown. They were like jigsaw puzzles half undone or with the pieces jumbled up.

It was often difficult to get close to them. They put up frail walls to protect themselves, for fear of being invaded, for fear of suffering. The better to hide their generous, wounded hearts.

# 36

Sunday. Today we are allowed to sleep in until 9.00. What a sad luxury! It makes no difference to me.

The morning is devoted to a make-up activity. I can't stand make-up. It irritates my eyes and skin, and it runs. I don't see the point of it. I want to be naturally beautiful, not to hide my defects. I want to be me, to be appreciated for who I am. I have never worn make-up, except to go to dances and that was awful because you had to wear a lot or it wouldn't show.

I don't know why, but I like the feeling of the brush stroking my face. It caresses me, it feels nice: I don't like cosmetics or wearing make-up but I like having my face made up.

It takes up the whole morning. According to the nurses I should make an effort to 'externalise' a bit more.

# 37

Lunch.

I spend the afternoon watching *Pretty Woman* with Manu. It is a video tape that was in with the books. It passes the time. I think it has been overrated.

What bothers me most about the TV room is the revolting smell of stale cigarettes – I can hardly bear to breathe in. When the film has finished I promise myself I will never set foot in the room again.

Mum comes in the evening – at the usual time. She has brought my 11-year-old sister Marion, which I'm not bothered about as I am completely indifferent to other people's presence or absence. She gives me communion. And some books she bought at a jumble sale a friend of hers organised. I am glad. They will keep me occupied for a while.

We talk. We say nothing. Goodbye.

# 38

Monday. I weigh 41 kilos. I feel rather proud of the progress I have made. I meet Dr Crapaud who tells me the nutritionist and the endocrinologist will be coming to see me. The endocrinologist is the doctor who will find out whether or not there is a medical reason for my depression and my 'shocking' physical condition.

In the afternoon I discover the pathetic theatre workshop: make a circle, hold hands and pass the ball of energy round, do the frog.

# 39

The days go by one after the other.

They take another blood sample for the endocrinologist to look at. Later on he comes to see me. He examines me with a cold stethoscope and takes my blood pressure (I love this but they hardly ever do it here) and he asks a lot of questions about my body and the illnesses I have had. He goes away saying everything looks normal, but that he will see when he gets the results of the blood tests. The others are amazed by all this medical attention (blood samples, visits from the doctor, ECG) – apparently it's unusual. In fact, they aren't equipped to treat anorexics here. Lucky I am not anorexic, then, just depressive, or so they tell me.

The following day, Tuesday, the others have gone on the monthly outing to St-Tropez. I am still too weak to go with them. I read the books Mum brought.

The man with the menus comes round in the morning. I smile to myself, thinking that tomorrow I will be the only one who has chosen my meals. I am also the only one who has seen the ward being cleaned. I am the only one who is left alone. It is frustrating always being alone, never seeing any doctors, psychologists or psychometricians. They keep telling me it's so I have time to think about the causes of my depression. They are wrong! It is unbearable brooding over your problems all day long, trying to make sense of them. As if they made any sense! When you are too submerged in a problem you don't have the distance to analyse it. On the contrary, you become even more bogged down; the more I think about my life the more worthless I feel. My fate is to suffer without ever knowing happiness. Why do sin and suffering outlive fleeting moments of joy?

I spent whole days searching for the causes of my depression. I found none. Each time I relived those painful moments of people's indifference, their insensitive words, their incomprehension and failure to help me, I hurt myself more. I went round in circles because no one listened to me or helped me discover which thread I needed to pull on in order to begin unravelling my tangled memories. I went over it all again and again in my mind until I became desperate, and I told myself nothing had any meaning and I should give up.

When I was getting nowhere or when I was in too much pain, I prayed. I offered my despair and suffering to God for the good of the world. The knowledge that He at least was listening to me, and the idea that my suffering wouldn't be in vain, gave me strength. I prayed a lot when I was in hospital...

In the afternoon I meet the nutritionist who gives me a chart showing the calorie contents of different foods. She explains to me what a balanced meal is and which nutritional needs correspond to my age group. She asks me whether there is any particular food I like that might stimulate my appetite. I tell her a man comes round every day and we choose what we want. She suggests we change my breakfast menu, which up until now has consisted of two soft rolls, two pieces of butter, a small pot of jam and a fruit juice. I ask for normal bread, as the rolls are too rubbery.

# 40

Wednesday. I weigh 41.3 kilos. I have put on a whole 500 grams! I feel very proud of my performance and I tell Dr Crapaud when I see her. All she can think of to say in her soft little voice with her big staring eyes is that I am still very weak, and that I will be in hospital 'for a good while yet'...

I cannot believe it! She has crushed my enthusiasm. I hate her silky-smooth voice that seems afraid of saying anything comforting. Her words pierce my heart like knives. I was full of hope, I was getting better. I wanted to live, to keep trying, and with one blow she knocks me down and tramples on me with her overly soft voice. If I could, right now, I would throw up all the antidepressant she has prescribed. She rubs my nose in all my mistakes: I haven't been good like the other children who do as they are told and eat their food. She hurls my futile efforts in my face like so many insults to my endeavours.

I begin a drastic diet there and then to try to purge myself as quickly as possible. I desperately want to prove to her how stupid and impotent she is.

I go back to my room and cry all morning.

That afternoon I discover the story-telling workshop. It calms me down slightly. Someone begins reading a story and then stops at a critical moment and the others make up an ending. One story is about a bear that has lost its mother, another about a warrior who must save his tribe, and a third about some children who have to change the seasons back. We take turns telling our endings. Not everyone has an imagination but almost no one refuses to take part. In fact, I am amazed by the sensitivity of these fiercely proud teenagers who, like the children they still are, listen to these stories as though they were a soothing balm nursing their sorrows one by one.

# 41

Thursday. Mum visits me again. She comes almost every other day. I am seeing the hospital chaplain, Father Philippe, today as well.

We are sitting in the canteen when he arrives, and everyone is surprised to see him, including me as I have never met him before. He has taken the stairs in order to come and fetch me, despite having what looks to me like a very bad leg. I feel touched and slightly guilty and I mention this as we leave, the others staring after us in disbelief.

After a long and difficult descent we reach the courtyard and he leads me over to the chapel. I don't remember the inside very well: two huge wooden doors opening onto a run-down interior and an old-fashioned high altar. We say a short prayer and go into the sacristy, where a table and some chairs are surrounded by cupboards crammed with objects – judging from all the glass bottles and papers lying about.

Father Philippe tells me a little about himself and his church with its collapsed clock tower. I am happy to be here. I feel more at home than up there. I feel as though I have escaped and am enjoying a break from hospital life. It is good to be far away from the ward in this reassuring, dusty old place, talking to a priest who doesn't look at me as if I were a specimen in the way the doctors and others do.

I confess and receive forgiveness. I feel safe. God is the only person to whom I have always dared show myself.

Then it is my turn to talk. Poor Father Philippe! It can't have been much fun for him. He had trouble understanding some of my words. He sensed it was difficult for me to talk about food, and was conscious of my ambivalence about my appearance. He assured me that depression was not a sin but a sign of true suffering, and that I must try to get better, to look at the positive side of life. He also told me I must eat or I would be unable to live, which is what God had created me for.

'I know it is difficult, but if you don't eat you won't have the strength to climb back up the slope. No matter what you do, whether you are fat or thin you will always be as God created you. You will always be you.'

Later on, whenever I felt bad or I didn't want to eat, I repeated those words to myself again and again. No. I cannot change anything. I will always be me.

Father Philippe walks me back to the ward. The others are already eating. They look as surprised as they did when we left. I sit down next to them and they start firing questions at me.

'Who was that guy you were with?' Fabien demands.

'He's a priest.'

'Do you really believe in God?' Léon is amazed.

'Yes.'

'I only wish I could. It's so hard! How can I believe in God if I can't see him? Do you know what I mean?' Zoë sighs, visibly perplexed.

'I can't see Him either. But I know He's there and it gives me strength. I know He will always love me. Even if everyone else abandons me. And I need that!'

'Do you pray here in hospital? How do you pray?'

They all seem so surprised. I am pleased they are listening to me and even more pleased to be able to talk about my faith. I explain.

'But what are you?' Manu asks. 'I mean, what's your religion? Christian?'

'Yes. I'm a Catholic.'

'I did the catechism up until primary school, but then I stopped . . . ,' Zoë says.

'So did I, with my grandma,' Fabien cuts in.

After a while some of them have had enough of religion! Zoë says she wants to talk to me about it again another time. I will talk to her about God and she will nickname me 'the voice of wisdom'. Soon they will all call me by my nickname, as if I knew the answer to everything!

# 42

Dr Crapaud has done me much harm. I can no longer force myself to eat and I sink back into despair. I really believed I would be able to leave here quickly. That I could cure myself through my own efforts sooner than they said. I watch all my hopes go up in smoke and I don't understand why they want to stop me from believing I might be happy again. I really don't understand anything about this place.

I also have the feeling they keep a closer watch on me than on the others – they are less trustful – and they listen to what I say as if it were baby-talk. They never try to understand they just nod and say, 'Yes, yes,' and pretend they are listening, in order to calm me.

I really am fed up. More than ever with food, hospital, people, but also with life and with myself. How could I have been so stupid as to believe them? It is impossible to be freely happy on earth. You have to be happy the way they want you to be. But my uniqueness is sacred to me.

I go and curl up on my bed, desperately miserable, betrayed by life and by others, no longer knowing who I am, and I cry my heart out.

I have tried to find answers, but I can't. When I was little I didn't have many friends. I did all I could to be accepted. I stopped playing with dolls because it was 'uncool'. I gave my Playmobil to my brothers and sisters because it was for babies. I won at marbles but it didn't win me any friends. I realised that I wouldn't be happy by trying to please other people and I distanced myself from them. I went through school feeling bad about myself. I had a few real friendships but my need for absolutes was so strong that they invariably ended in pain and disappointment or died natural deaths. All the same I was happy there. And then, because I was alone, I decided to try to find happiness by sacrificing myself to a cause: my beliefs. And I ended up making myself ill. I can't relate to other people's values and my own make me suffer.

And now when I finally change my position and decide to live and eat, Dr Crapaud rubs my nose in my failures. Why! Why! Why!

I keep coming to the same conclusion – I have nothing to do on this earth.

# 43

The same day, Thursday. Since yesterday I have lost every gram I had put on, and in two days' time I will weigh 38 kilos. Dr Crapaud rejected me just when I was beginning to open up to others. I thought she would help me and instead she pushed me away. I sink back into despair, allowing myself to waste away.

I can feel the others staring at me, but it doesn't upset me any more. I am numb, wrapped in a protective fog, impervious to the outside world. I am alone with my pain. I have closed the door, no longer letting others in, no longer listening to them for fear of suffering even more. And I allow myself to drift, utterly alone, on the turbulent seas of the ward. I am back where I started.

When I think of my time in the hospital these are the things I remember, and which make me feel bad because I still don't understand. I hear Skyrock radio playing, the sound of shouting and crying. I relive the intense silence, the cold. I smell the odour of clean floors and fragrant lavender, the ice-cold or burning-hot food, the aloe-vera shower gel. I see the shabby white, green, beige and colourless walls. The faces lost in deep despair, the concerned or strict-looking nurses. And I see me, not loving myself, a lifeless zombie in that shadow world. And I experience the same feeling of discomfort, of suffocation, as if someone were pressing down on my chest and trying to stop me from breathing.

# 44

Friday. I was quite happy to join in the arts and crafts farce again today, but this time the nurses try to show me where I'm going wrong.

Dr Crapaud calls me to her office simply to tell me that I risk being put on a drip, and that I will stay here as long as I continue refusing to eat. I despise her unspeakably soppy, cute little office. I have been waiting for this. I dare them to put me on a drip.

# 45

I am still not eating, I am letting myself die. I feel that I am closer to freedom, and I tell myself that I will never have known happiness. And I cry.

The anti-depressant was a strange thing. I wouldn't exactly say I was addicted to it. I never accepted taking it and I always denied its power. The only effect it had on me was to stop me from thinking: my thoughts went fuzzy, as if the grey filter through which I usually saw the world had been tinted orange or dark red. It was just an illusion, and I could no longer see anything. In any case, it didn't give me back my appetite or my will to live. It just robbed me of myself a little more.

# 46

I need someone else, someone from outside who will believe me. I remember my godmother. Mum gives me her number and I ring her.

I waited eagerly for her call every evening, like a rest at the end of a long day. She was frank with me. She told me I must try to get better, and that she was worried about me, instead of dutifully, or politely, enquiring after my health like other people, or saying nothing for fear of hurting me. It is their pained, awkward expressions that kill me; they don't have the courage to understand me. Maybe they are afraid of suffering. But I need honesty.

I don't know whether my godmother helped me in starting to eat again or in my struggle with myself, but feeling she loved and understood me and wasn't trying to convince me I was wrong was a comfort to me. She was simply there for me, and that was what I needed: to know I still mattered to somebody.

# 47

The comings and goings on the ward continue. A boy of Russian extraction with a strong accent climbs aboard our drifting raft. The good thing about hospital is that there is no need to explain the rules of the game to anyone. As soon as they walk through the door they understand, or rather they endure without understanding. It is not the new arrival who asks the questions but the others who interrogate him. In short, he updates the usual topics of conversation.

However, we respect his silence. It echoes our own thoughts. Emptiness is what we have in common. This boy doesn't seem unhappy though, and he has soon lost his shyness and is laughing with Léon. He even calls us 'slutskys'. Three days later he is gone. We never knew why he was here.

Saturday. The activities follow their preset programme. In arts and crafts we make decorations for the Christmas meal on 19 December. I busy myself painting, modelling and cutting out angels and nativity figures though I know I won't be here for the meal as this is a short-stay ward. The nurses exclaim over my capable fingers – which doesn't matter to me one way or the other.

I now weigh 38 kilos! I have lost 15 kilos since the summer. Dr Crapaud lays the blame on the dosage of my anti-depressant, and increases it. I realise I am a minor in the eyes of the world and I let myself be manipulated, refusing to allow the situation to continue by depriving myself of food.

Mum visits me and as usual I am absent before, during and after her visits. She speaks to me and I reply, as though filling the silence were a game. It passes the time. Yet I get so little out of it that I wouldn't be able to say what we talked about, or even whether Dad came or not. I remember once Mum bringing me some perfume. It was a gift from a friend of hers who came with us on the pilgrimage to Bosnia-Herzegovina. I was deeply touched. Giving something that belongs to us, however small, is an act of self-sacrifice, and I found it hard to believe I could be worthy of such a gesture. In this sense, I still attach a lot of importance to gifts. For me, even a postcard is a beautiful gift because it means someone is thinking of me. This is why I was pleased when Mum chose and bought those clothes for me. She did it for me. It seemed completely unthinkable at the time!

Since I have been allowed to receive calls some of my teachers have rung me. I tell them how everything is going and say yes when they ask me anxiously whether I am feeling any better. I feel touched when I hear their voices: I haven't been completely forgotten outside this place. But none of my friends (I didn't really have any) or classmates have phoned.

# 48

Since the Crapaud incident, I have been spending even more time thinking. I am too weak to do my exercises properly (and anyway it is too risky now that I am sharing with Fleur), and I don't feel like sleeping or being with the others: given that we all think about the same things I might as well spare myself their futile thoughts by keeping mine to myself.

Sunday. They are taking us bowling today. Even me! I have never been before. We find ourselves in a large hall. It is almost empty. I like it here. We take turns trying to knock the skittles over. Fleur is the best at it. I take their advice and use the lighter balls, but they still feel heavy to me. I don't do too badly, though. Just as we are getting in the cars to leave, a boy rides up on a scooter. It is Fleur's boyfriend. She has arranged for him to come and meet us at the exit. I am so happy for her and glad she has been able to score a small victory against that miserable hospital.

My second weekend here is over. Will they carry out their threat and put me on a drip? This interminable weekend brings home to me the reality of being in hospital – as if that were necessary. I have to get out of here. This can't go on. I am tired of being seen as irresponsible. I must submit to their rules, to the tyranny of food, in order to win my freedom.

When I realise they aren't going to put me on a drip, I give in to pressure and force myself to eat. This food that I don't want passes through my body. I put it in my mouth and force myself to swallow, but I still don't accept it. I make no effort to change this.

I won't put on any weight for several days.

# 49

Monday. I see the psychologist again: the same scenario as last time. She attempts to understand my life, my family, my way of thinking. When I tell her I stopped going to school in order to come into hospital she congratulates me. She thinks it was because I wanted to devote myself to getting better. In fact, I was burning my bridges. I gave up on life long before coming in here.

I also see the psychometrician. She explains to me that her treatment is based on corporal therapy: if I feel good physically I will improve mentally. I am willing to believe her, especially since my mind is completely cut off from this body it detests. She talks to me about modelling, drawing, playing with hoops or balls, and gymnastics. We spend the first session 'getting to know each other'. I am already looking forward to the second session. This will turn out, pointlessly, to be the day before I am discharged.

# 50

Tuesday. They certainly succeeded in making me eat. I gave in but I still haven't put on any weight and so I am still not allowed on the Tuesday outing.

I am going to see Dr Crapaud to tell her I have started eating again, and to make her understand that I must leave here. I am sure she won't listen as I am not putting on any weight, but I am curious to see whether her attitude has changed. Of course it hasn't and she puts me down exactly as before. I thought as much, and it confirms what I already knew: I can only count on myself.

I am finding hospital more and more unbearable. I decide to make an extra effort so they will allow me home for the weekend. I have a few days left until then. I must get out of this place. I feel as if I only came in here to be examined, like a culture in a Petri dish which is hardly ever opened for fear of introducing infection (like help, for example). Dr Crapaud only made me come here so she could control my antidepressant, or rather *her* vile antidepressant, so she could say she did her duty as a good psychiatrist.

I only wanted to be happy, but I am not allowed to be myself in here after all. I feel bitterly betrayed. I can no longer trust her.

I MUST get out. I have to, for the simple reason that I can't stand it in here any longer. Once again I make up my mind to try to put on some weight; I can always lose it after I leave. I keep remembering Father Philippe's words: 'No matter what you do, whether you are fat or thin, you will always be as God created you. You will always be you.'

I hope that happiness is waiting for me outside.

# 51

I feel slightly more sociable, but I am incapable of thinking at all. The world makes no sense to me.

Claire and Léon are in love. Fleur ran away and was brought back by the police. She rings her boyfriend every day and he comes to the courtyard to see her. She signals to him through the bars on the windows. I am complicit in their secret and pretend to be talking to her whenever a nurse comes in: visits from non-family members are forbidden, as are mobile phones.

The Russian boy is replaced by Damien, a diabetic who sleeps all day and plays video games all night. He doesn't seem in such a bad way either. Only now he is here in hospital he spends all day in his room.

As for me, I keep trying, though I find it very hard. I manage to put on 200 grams and so on Friday I am allowed to go to the supermarket with four other teenagers and the nurse who is going to buy a birthday cake for one of the cleaners, a very sweet little old lady who is going to be 60. It is a small victory. However, they continue watching me like hawks.

That same week I attempt to renew my contact with civilisation. I write to people in my class to see if they will reply, I ring a girl I was friends with at primary school, and I write to some other friends. It keeps me busy and makes me feel as though I am getting better.

# 52

I am allowed home for the weekend! Mum comes and fetches me at 10.00. I am making a model when she arrives and the nurses show her my 'work'. I am in a hurry to leave.

The weekend is terrifying. I am plunged from the cold, empty silence of the ward into an over-heated house where I feel I have never belonged. My brothers and sisters crowd round me as if I were the Messiah, wanting to know everything. I am caught off guard, unable to speak. I am not even pleased to see them. They make me nervous swarming all over me, and I feel very ill at ease and out of place. I know they only want to be friendly, to ask me how I am, and hear my news, but their insistent presence makes me feel faint, and I push past them avoiding their questions, and creep up the stairs to my room like a shadow. I lie down on my bed and cry.

Their initial interest gives way to the usual hubbub of weekends at home. Everyone squabbling and provoking each other. The shouting, running, slamming of doors and clattering of objects makes me dizzy.

I eat very little but it feels like a lot.

This Saturday, Mum and I are going to buy some make-up. I told her about the session with the nurses and how they think make-up suits me. In fact, I tell myself, this could be a way of convincing the hospital staff that I am getting better.

On Sunday morning we go to Mass, and I count the minutes until the evening. I cannot possibly live here.

Maxime and Marion catch the 3.30pm train and the house quietens down. But the relative silence is broken by the hubbub of the three youngest resuming their activities.

Mum suggests I relax in a hot bath. I take her advice and stretch out in the tub. But I have to get out again after five minutes: even with the buoyancy of the water, resting on my shoulders, my pelvis and heels is too painful; the bottom of the tub isn't soft like the mattress I spend my life lying on.

I climb into the car feeling relieved, knowing what awaits me, but above all glad to be leaving all this behind.

I have a peaceful night, almost happy to be back at the hospital.

# 53

I make my face up very clumsily. I imagine I must look quite funny half-covered in the stuff! And this mirror I can hardly recognise myself in only adds to the difficult job of making myself look pretty. Not to mention the cheap make-up we bought which doesn't go on easily... The nurses applaud when I emerge from the bathroom looking like a clown. I have the double impression of no longer being me: I am what people want me to be. I stop the make-up farce after three days. It bores me.

I am making progress.

# 54

This week I am allowed on the Tuesday outing. I watch the others play football with Claire, who is smoking.

Fleur preferred to stay behind at the hospital. She wanted to be alone and do some cooking. When we come back there is a pile of pancakes waiting for us in the canteen. I don't eat any but the others pounce on them and devour the lot. Fleur, who didn't want any at tea-time, comes back later to find they haven't even left one for her. She tries to hide her anger and disappointment, but it shows on her face.

I don't know why this moment has stayed with me. I even remember there was cherry jam, sugar and chestnut purée. Maybe it is because we were doing something 'normal': enjoying squabbling, and eating food that wasn't in plastic trays.

# 55

Anastacia arrives. She is a sick girl. Very thin. She is 'euphoric' and doesn't realise what she is doing. Apparently she mistakes her fantasies for reality: she believes she is a queen who must be obeyed and she might even jump out of the window, thinking she can fly. It seems to me the nurses are very hard on her.

Anastacia often screams at them when they ask her something. She flies into rages and lashes out. More than once they have locked her in the room that I have never been in at the end of the ward. It is where they put people to calm them down. She bangs on the door, shouting incoherently. Then the nurses, helped by Karim, strap her down and inject her with sedatives. A heavy silence descends upon us and we look at one another, bewildered, shocked, frightened and confused, before going back to our rooms, hardly daring to disturb the quiet of the corridor by speaking, and not wanting to be overheard by the nurses.

Fleur also flew into a rage one day and they gave her an injection. Only one. Anastacia hardly ever comes out. I must have seen her three times. She is definitely strange, but I would never have thought she was mad if no one had told me.

We talk about it later amongst ourselves. And about our prospects when we leave hospital. Freedom, a bad job, another hospital – a long-stay one this time. And our hopes. Finding a long-lost father, gaining a mother's love, seeing a little brother cured, getting through school! I feel distant from them. My case is so much more simple and yet so complicated. Nothing outside of me can help because this only concerns me. Me and my ideals.

I demand too much from life: the world must change for me to be happy. I don't have any real problems. I am good at everything: school, dancing, drawing, singing. I feel touched that my fellow castaways don't hold this against me, or despise me for it. I am their equal because I suffer too. When I feel lost they draw me into their circle, they accept me – regardless of how different we are. And I am grateful.

They try to help one another, to understand and find solutions. I am here for them. I offer them my support and they do the same for me.

They are often angry with their parents. One girl's mother blames her for the stretch marks she got during pregnancy. 'She wanted to have me, dammit! So she should take the consequences. She's like a kid! And she's supposed to be the grown-up!' The girl bursts into tears. We put our arms round one another and find relief in letting go.

I try to put their minds at rest; I wasn't nicknamed 'the voice of wisdom' for nothing!

It's a shame the voice won't work for me.

# 56

I am slowly beginning to calm down, to relax. I feel less irritable. Not that I like being in hospital. Nobody likes being somewhere they don't feel at home. But since I've been with the others I have realised I am not alone and, more importantly, I can get through this. It all depends on me. I need to accept things the way they are without wanting to change them. Or myself. This means loving myself, and it is the most difficult part. Mum is always saying to me, 'I love you,' which is exactly why I don't believe her.

Zoë once asked me to say to her, 'God loves you.' It is easy: it is one of the only things I am certain of. I placed my hands on her shoulders, looked deep into her eyes, and said, 'God loves you.' She was happy. She says it sounds true when I say it. I wish someone would say to me, 'I love you. Life is beautiful.' But it is not something I can ask.

# 57

Wednesday. Nina arrives. She cuts her wrists her first night here. I know exactly how she feels!

Like me she has no real reason to be depressed. Does there need to be a reason? People are unhappy mostly by default, because they don't have enough to be happy about.

Nina sings – not 'in public', but to herself, or to me when we are alone in her room or mine. Never in front of the nurses. She is a fan of Lara Fabian, and sings her songs beautifully.

I often spend time with her for the simple pleasure of hearing her sing. She talks to me too. She would like to make a career in music, to live off her singing. She seems to have it all worked out: the name Nina is no good because there is a singer in Germany called Nena.

She is my age. Of Spanish extraction. She has dark, curly hair and a penetrating gaze that should be intense but is suddenly weakened by a surge of emotion which fills her eyes with tears.

Something draws me to her. She is confused and unhappy, and yet alive. She can be cured. Maybe this is why I am drawn to her. I want her to be cured. I want to prove to myself that it is possible to be cured. I want to help her, to be a sort of big sister by explaining the hospital rules to her. Though I realise she doesn't need me in order to understand them. Everything here is so easy and at the same time so difficult.

I think she gets on better with Fleur and Claire anyway. I am happy just to tag along, the only difference being that I feel closer to the other two girls now that Nina is here.

I have always liked singing. But I soon stopped because I didn't want to disturb the others who felt there was already enough noise in the house. I couldn't sing at school as I wasn't in the choir. Also, I had been nicknamed 'Castafiore' (after the opera singer from the *Tintin* books) because of my 'high-pitched' voice. I assumed it was also because I sang badly, out of tune and had a screechy voice. I was gradually bullied into keeping quiet.

But when I hear Nina singing so beautifully and with such feeling, it makes me believe I can sing again too. If it won't disturb the others. If I have the courage.

One day I do have the courage. I ask Nina what she thinks of my singing. We shut ourselves in the bathroom (the ideal place because it has a lock on the door) and we talk. We share our thoughts. Not just blurting out words that only strike a chord if they refer to suffering, like with the others. Music and singing – her singing, which I admire – are what bring us together. She sings for me, and I have never heard such a beautiful voice.

Then it is my turn. I feel very awkward. I want to do my best so that she won't regret listening to me and I feel a flicker of hope that she might like my singing. But my voice catches in my throat, and I sing in a weak voice, self-conscious because I know someone is listening. I give a pitiful rendering of 'San Francisco' by Maxime le Forestier, conscious of having chosen the wrong song because it doesn't suit my voice and is too old-fashioned.

Humiliated, I hurriedly finish the first verse and with it my recital of one of the only non-religious songs I know.

I am afraid to meet her gaze, which is no longer that of a fellow depressive but of a teacher judging my performance. She tells me, earnestly, that I have a pretty voice, but that I need to work on my breathing and learn to use my stomach muscles, and that I must practise. I don't know if she really means it, but her words give me a glimmer of hope. For her part, I think knowing that someone listens to and appreciates her voice, and shows an interest in her passion, does her as much good.

I dream of her bringing out a CD and my writing the lyrics to a song for her. She is touched, and I am glad I have made her happy.

We spend a lot more time together, especially us girls: we listen to Nina sing or watch Fleur do acrobatics; we hold each other when we are cold or need comforting. These are good times. Suffering can bring people together. And sometimes, when one of us confides in the others, we break up the gathering out of respect for that person's intimacy. As if their words should be left floating in the air awaiting further reflection, or allowed to fall gently to the ground like dead leaves, not troubled by having any other words on top.

# 58

Thursday. Léon is discharged. He is not cured but he seems better – he has desires, projects. Claire is the next person to leave the hospital. But she isn't well at all. I thought people only left here when they were 'better'. Claire is crying when she leaves, miserable, overwhelmed with despair. I feel devastated.

So, we are just left here not knowing whether we will ever get better! This is fine for the lucky ones but what about the others? No. I can't believe this. After Claire has left, Dr Crapaud calmly explains to us that we aren't discharged because we are cured, but because we are 'on the right track'. That's such a euphemism: she ought to have been a politician!

I promise myself I won't let her sweep me under the carpet: a problem which is diagnosed and left untreated is far more dangerous than one which is left undiagnosed. My problem has been identified. I won't allow myself to be destroyed.

# 59

Friday. Zoë leaves in the morning and Fabien in the evening. Both for the long-stay hospital. This wasn't their first time in the short-stay hospital which is only for stays of up to one month.

I am finding it hard to let go of my beliefs and principles. But the fact that I have started eating again helps me progress. Winning one small battle can feel like a huge victory – especially when the enemy is you. I have no appetite and I am forcing myself to eat again through sheer willpower – not so that Dr Crapaud will be lenient with me or allow me to leave, but to show I can beat her, that I don't need her, and that she should never have put me in hospital.

# 60

The end of my third week in hospital. At last I have put on some weight, about 100 grams. You have no idea how hard it was. It took me more than four days just to put on 100 grams. Four days of constant discomfort, of feeling continually divided between rejoicing whenever I succeeded in swallowing more than a mouthful, and being inwardly tormented by the idea. I even worked out a way of using up energy lying on the bed reading.

I have regained some of my strength through eating. And my stomach is slowly beginning to hurt less. I no longer feel so reluctant to sit down to meals, and although eating is still difficult mealtimes have become almost friendly occasions again – despite the setting.

Eating more food, more regularly, gives me the energy I need to help me improve. I know I am making progress because I am no longer constantly on the alert wondering whether my blood sugar is low or thinking ahead to the firm, strong-minded attitude I must adopt at the next meal. I no longer need to convince myself how repulsive the food on my plate looks (even though here it is true) in order to persuade myself not to eat it. The fact is, in the beginning food only disgusted me because I managed to make myself disgusted by it.

Now I am eating again I think about all these processes, about all the negative feelings food inspired in me, and I tell myself that using force is never good. Of course each case is different, but forcing people can make them shut themselves off – sometimes forever – because they are afraid of suffering even more from the violence you want to inflict on them.

# 61

As I improve so my thinking progresses. I am too much of a perfectionist. I feel this need to throw myself completely into everything I do. It was the same with my belief in purity, only it led to my downfall. I rejected the world and its contradictions. The hospital left me to my own devices, which could have hastened my end by making me reject the world even more. But I am a 'fighter': 'mighty in battle'. I won't let myself be destroyed, especially without knowing why. I resisted, refusing to allow them to control me, to bury me in that psychiatric hospital. I was determined to leave, to fight my way out using every last gram of strength I had left.

'Fight' is not a word I use lightly. It can mean a lot of things, but for me it refers to the tensing up of my entire being, mind and body, when I need to resist the temptation to give up completely. This can be very difficult, impossible even, when you have no goal. In hospital my aim was to fight against my incarceration; I added freedom to my ideal of purity. Finding myself in a worse situation than before, and above all one I hadn't chosen to be in, awoke in me a sort of 'instinct for freedom', like the instinct to survive.

I fought Dr Crapaud to prove to her I was healthy. Like the others she didn't believe me. She knocked me down and trampled on me. So I rebelled against her and her decision to continue keeping me in hospital. I could have refused to play the game and discharged myself, but this would have been an admission of failure and weakness. My honour was at stake and I wasn't about to give in. I forced myself to swallow food and keep it down, to accept myself as I was through sheer willpower in the same way I had convinced myself I was useless.

In reality, deep down, what helped me keep going was the hope that somebody would come along and prove to me that my beliefs had given me a distorted view of life. I hadn't decided to die, only to wait for death to come. It is not the same thing. Luckily someone listened to me when I was about to let go, which proves it is never too late. Someone from outside, who had a more objective view of things: Father Philippe. His words guided me.

My eyes are fixed straight ahead on the light at the end of the tunnel: I have to leave here at any cost. In order to be able to eat, I tell myself that refusing food has made me weak and stopped me from helping others and doing good.

I want Nina to get better too. I hope she won't have to stay in here.

I have been here long enough now. I admit that I am feeling better, quite well even, compared to when I first arrived. This is no thanks to the hospital, in any case not to the doctors.

# 62

We are only depressive because we lack something: love, success, friends. We need help re-educating ourselves to appreciate life. More than anything we need guiding, like little children who refuse to go on walking until someone takes their hand. We need patient help in order to rediscover the world in a different light, to savour life's beauty and fill the emptiness left by our need, our refusal and our indifference until we are bursting with joy and happiness. It takes determination to reach this state. It doesn't happen overnight. There can come a point when our suffering is too great, and we are unable to fight any more. This is when we most need help from others.

I only wish someone had said to me, 'Life is beautiful and I love you.'

Nobody did.

And yet isn't this the first thing you would say to someone who is suffering?

# 63

Friday evening. I am impatient to achieve my goal. It will be like a moment of truth when all my theories are put to the test. Will I accept the world? I dream of being in harmony with everyone. I can't wait to live, to prove myself.

# 64

My second weekend at home is nothing like my first. I feel like laughing, and I look for any opportunity, barely able to contain my joy. I am eager to answer my brothers' and sisters' questions, but they no longer seem to feel the need to ask me any – I think they were hurt and worried by my silence last weekend. I regret not having listened when they were giving me their full attention. It feels like a missed opportunity.

I have to say I find it very irritating when people ask me to tell them about the hospital. There is nothing to *tell*. People in hospital suffer because they are cut off from others; they are deprived of oxygen and have none to give, and their conversations often take place in silence or consist of listening to another's monologue.

For my part, I am happy and relieved to see the life that still reigns in our house: the screams and laughter and running about make me feel at home. The world has waited for me, nothing has changed. Everyone lives exactly as they did before. I can try my luck again, like starting a new life. Only I must be careful not to spoil this one. I open my eyes and ears to everything around me, my senses are fully awake. I have never been so aware of the Christmas decorations, the smells in the street, the lights, people's faces, the food we eat.

I feel the contrast between the times when I denied my

own life and these moments of euphoria when everything is meaningful again. Even though nothing has changed for the others – indeed *because* nothing has changed for them – life is there for me to rediscover, and from now on I look carefully at everything around me in search of newness, beauty and joy. I am hungry for life. I am constantly restless and need to be out of doors – as if I had to catch up on all the sensations and discoveries I have missed by being in hospital. I wear everyone out but have an endless supply of energy.

I long for the moment when I will finally be discharged. In fact, I think of nothing else. I feel at home here, happy to be me. I realise I am still too thin and need to put on more weight. This was driven home to me when I tried on some of my old clothes and found they were still baggy. But I am in no hurry to put on weight. I want to let life in slowly, not all at once, like making a mayonnaise, adding the oil drop by drop so the egg doesn't separate. I have regained my confidence, and with it the power to wait. I know I am going to be all right.

I enjoy my weekend at home.

I return to the hospital feeling calm – knowing I will be leaving soon.

# 65

I am entering my fourth and final week. I submit to all the hospital rules without any fuss. I even eat well. I am in a good mood. In short: I am ready. I know it is only a question of time now. I really do feel better.

The weekend was a great relief to me: I enjoyed being with the members of my family instead of ignoring them or only focusing on their bad sides, selfishly thinking about how they might hurt me. And I appreciated my Mum's cooking. I passed the test: I am qualified for life on the outside. I am happy, though a little disappointed that I had to wait this long, a little frustrated not to be out already. If only they had helped me instead of leaving me to go through it on my own.

I discover a new sensation: appetite. In this case you could even call it hunger. It has to be said that as I am 15 kilos underweight and living in this under-heated hospital it is hardly surprising if food seems to call to me. The taste of freedom I had at the weekend has fuelled my appetite for life, and I want to be healthy. I am hungry for new sensations. Taste itself is like a forgotten experience for me. I so successfully convinced myself that food was bad for me that it lost all its flavour; I transformed smells into nauseating stenches that disgusted me to the point of making me want to be sick, despite my empty stomach!

So I doubly appreciate meals now: I savour the food and

I feel my strength surging back. Each mouthful is a step closer to freedom, like thrusting a sword deeper and deeper into the weakening enemy. I even manage to eat up everything in the hospital trays, which are big, and to enjoy the bland, overcooked hospital food: the unripe fruit, the rock-hard cakes, the oily pasta, the meat dissolving in its unvarying sauce, the vegetables that all look alike, the watery soup... As I have eaten practically nothing for months this food doesn't put me off. As if I were discovering what it means to eat.

# 66

I smile, I feel good, but I keep myself to myself. Other hopeless cases have arrived since our group of walking wounded left. I would like to be able to help them, and to be able to help Nina too. Occasionally I go and see them, but mostly I stay in my room. It is really important for me to get to know myself again. Unfortunately, the others don't always understand this – especially not the nurses. Of course they can see I am getting better – I even told them so. At first they didn't believe me, but now I know I have won them over.

It is difficult to have any privacy here. People tend to barge in just when you are beginning to enjoy being in peace. They generally mean well: 'Come along, you poor thing, you mustn't stay all by yourself. Come and join us, you'll be less bored!' The poor things don't realise they are disturbing my calm and concentration, which are the exact opposite of boredom, and that being alone suits me very well. It is not a sign of madness or a rejection of the world. I just need time to find my bearings. Once I am at peace with myself I shall be able to communicate more and better with everything and everyone around me.

Of course it's up to you if you want me to stay with you 24 hours a day, spraying you with my poison because I need to let everything inside me burst out in an uncontrollable flood! I really am too confused, mentally, to be completely sociable. It is better for me to take the time to organise my thoughts before I open my mouth. And holding forth in complete freedom is so much more relaxing. I find talking just to say uninteresting or nonsensical things so pointless that during my 'meditation breaks' I analyse the effect of what I say and what others say to me. Given the confused flow of my unpredictable thoughts, I am hoping this way to make more sense when I speak: you have to be so careful not to hurt people, especially when they are as fragile as they are here in this hospital...

When it is not the other teenagers it is the nurses who worry about you being on your own. I should add that now I sense I am on the road to recovery I love to think about the happy life I am going to have after I leave the hospital: I am like a baby still in the womb knowing I am about to be born, and preparing myself for my future life and projects. I really do have 'my whole life ahead of me'. Anything is possible.

Actually, I am more like an adult about to be born than a child: I have already lived a little and suffered a lot. I know the world – you remember, that little creature I tried to starve to death. I am excited to meet him again – like an old adversary I have fought with for so long he has become a part of me. I am eager to see how we will get on.

I also want to rejoin the girl guides, and I spend hours inventing new games, new excursions, new menus that will be a change from the usual routine. I am already looking forward to the next summer camp. For me the guide movement represents friendship, self-improvement, self-reliance and respect for nature. I cling to this ideal, I think about it because it gives me an aim, something to keep me going on the path outside. I think ahead, I plan for hours at a time. I can't wait to sacrifice myself, to offer my good qualities and the results of all my thinking to others: I can't wait to share.

# 67

I am about to leave the hospital. But it is still just as important for me to analyse this. Why am I allowed to leave? Because I am getting better, of course. So what was wrong with me? I have always been *me* before, during and after my depression, so why this depression? They asked me this question again and again during four long weeks, and I was incapable of thinking about it, let alone finding any answers, because I was alone and blinded by my situation. I can stand back a little from my experience now and yet it is recent enough for me still to be able to feel all the emotions that overwhelmed me, and the effects of all the dogma they imposed on me. Whatever happens, I don't think I will ever forget how violent it was.

I decide to try to discover the reasoning that led me to withdraw into another world rather than look for the causes of my depression. I ask myself why I no longer wanted to live. It hurts. It is like admitting that I took a completely wrong turning, that I wilfully wasted part of my life. Today, those painful moments have become almost crystallised, hard and impenetrable. And however much they are shaken or banged about they can do no more harm because in a sense they have lost all feeling. That other me has vanished and nothing can hurt her now.

So what did happen then? In keeping with my ideals I wanted to become perfect, that is, to be a model example.

I had to achieve mastery in all the areas I had identified as representing the highest qualities: beauty, purity, kindness, generosity, endurance, patience, loyalty, concern for others, excellence in my studies as well as in everyday and household chores.

'Individual freedom ends where other people begin.' My freedom had no beginning because other people's began in its place. Everything I did revolved around others; my sole aim was to bring about a better world. I made myself pretty so I would be a pleasure for others to look at, a sort of visual feast; I wanted to be pure so that I would live up to my ideal and always show the good side of humanity to others to encourage them to improve themselves; I wanted to be kind, generous, diligent, patient and loyal in order to make life easier for others; I wanted to excel at school to please my parents but above all so that my school results would not be an extra source of worry to them. I also felt I had to please my teachers, to be a sort of inspiration to them as a pupil.

In a sense I programmed myself to take on other people's problems so as to make their lives easier, and to avoid being a problem myself. I tried to make myself small so as not to bother them. And I succeeded: I became so mechanical, so impersonal, so inhuman that people no longer noticed me. They stopped saying hello to me, as if by choosing self-denial I had ceased to exist. They collided with me as they would with an inanimate object, invisible in the dark. I remember when I first arrived at the hospital the others saying they were afraid of bumping into me in case I fell over. My physical frailty worried them. I had no substance, no presence: they had to be careful of me because they couldn't see me. I had succeeded so well in making myself small that I ended up disappearing.

What I refused to see was that disappearing would be painful. Strangely enough I had anticipated everything: I devised strategies, I planned in advance how I would respond to each fresh onslaught, each new temptation. I spent my life resigning myself, depriving myself: of games – of reading even – so I would have more time for others; of food so I would be beautiful in keeping with the demands of fleeting fashion; of singing so as not to disturb the others.

I filled my head with thoughts of a practical nature: what I needed to do to help others; how I could become more rigorous in my demands on myself and not forget crucial things like doing my homework. I was constantly tense, constantly vigilant. I could not allow myself to fail on any level. The only escape I had was during sleep.

The result of this relentless mental tyranny was psychological breakdown. Instead of making myself small I grew into a source of concern for my parents, until I ended up becoming their biggest problem. I was unable to accept this. My ideals could not lie. And yet it became increasingly difficult to deny the worried look on my parents' faces. When I saw how upset they were I felt guilty and stepped up my demands on myself. And I made things worse.

These were the basic workings of my depression: I had risked so much in return for so little! I had to wait until I was getting better in order to realise this, to see that it wasn't making me happy and was dangerous for me, to accept that it wasn't helping others and, worse still, it was causing them more problems! I was forced to admit that what they had been saying to me all along was true. I was mistaken.

I am what you might call lucid with regard to my painful past: I want to understand. And yet I feel no bitterness. I am not angry with anyone – not even with myself. A priest once said there are two ways of responding to past suffering: wanting to forget and resentment. For me there is a third way. I don't mind talking about it because it is part of who I am, and it is one of the things that influenced my recovery: I accepted myself as I was, including my whole past, from that very last weekend I spent at home onwards. Even though it wasn't yet past history. Even though it never will be past history.

Accepting yourself is a true challenge. Up till then I had submitted to the outside without letting any part of myself show through. This meant I could never relax. Most of all it stopped me, in my supremely important relationship with others, from allowing them to benefit from my good qualities: suffering had made me selfish. I must learn – or re-learn, which is more difficult – to open up to others. It makes me think of that person who has no friends. She goes 'begging' for friendship. She tries to please everyone. She is a puppet and has no personality of her own – nothing to offer. And people don't care about her, they aren't interested. Yet surely, on the contrary, in order for friendship to exist everyone must contribute their individuality to the group, like a 'breath of fresh air'. Through contributing something new and unique she will earn a place in the esteem and hearts of others. It is only by revealing and sharing my qualities that I will acquire my true worth. Otherwise I shall always be like a weather-cock, never at rest, constantly conforming to other people's desires even though I may not agree with them, so as not to be alone. Because being alone is bad in their eyes. I make up my mind to be myself. It will be so much easier! I will be so much more free to think and to act. I shan't need to worry any longer about my outward appearance. I shall simply be myself, serving others by allowing them to benefit from me.

Another challenge is the tyranny of physical appearance. In order to be thinner and thinner I deprived myself of food. And even though I was so accustomed to not eating that it was no longer a physical effort, mentally speaking I was constantly vigilant about renewing my feelings of disgust towards food. I practised a relentless, exhausting form of brainwashing on myself. The tyranny of appearance never really made me happy, then. By definition I could never be satisfied because I always needed to be thinner. If there had been nothing left of me but skin and bone I would still have wanted to be thinner. In the end how valuable you are to others depends on how much you value yourself.

# 68

A lot of people say to me that this kind of experience makes you stronger. I don't know whether that's true or not. Let's just say you come out of it enriched, with a fresh, clear vision of the world. I think you are only stronger when you truly conquer the enemy; only then do you feel strong enough to go and do battle with life's problems.

On the other hand, I disagree with the idea that you can know your limits. For this to be true you would need to know the root causes of the problem. I still don't know what caused my depression but I don't believe it is the most important question.

# 69

During the few days left between now and freedom, I spend a lot of time with the others. I have been thinking, 'making sure', in a way, that I was right when I said I was cured, and right to want to be cured.

There are a few new arrivals on the ward. I talk to them. I want some of my optimism to rub off on them so they won't end up going to 'long-stay' hospitals like Zoë and Fabien. Depression, unhappiness and pain seem so alien to me now. Everything I experience is heightened by my hunger for life.

I see my 'work' decorating the hall, like the feathers left by a bird that has flown its cage. The angels, the three wise men...

I talk a lot. I want to protect the new arrivals, to comfort them. At the same time I feel I am no longer really here. I have already left the hospital. I am in the decompression chamber, in the waiting room. As if I were the doctor.

# 70

I am waiting to leave.

On Tuesday evening they tell me that, as of tomorrow, I can push open the cage doors and fly away, at last.

I wait patiently. I savour every moment of my life – I have wasted so many! I also want to fix in my memory this atmosphere, this incomparable emptiness.

Mum arrives.

I say goodbye to everyone: to the nurses looking deceptively sad, to Dr Crapaud. I know this is how it was, though I don't remember.

I am outside. I am thinking only of what is to come – the hospital is over. I am bursting with energy and joy, despite the 10 kilos I still need to put on. For the moment all is well, and it will only get better. After winning a battle you feel invincible.

I climb into the car. We drive away from the hospital. I soak up everything around me. I am swept along on a tide of colours, sounds and sensations. I want to take in every little detail. I am brimming with joy.

It is light outside. It was dark when I arrived.

I feel as if I am waking up from a bad dream.

# Epilogue

The first thing I did when I arrived home was finish off a packet of chocolate biscuits that was lying on the table.

Dr Crapaud had recommended I go to boarding school in order to remove me somewhat from my 'traumatic family environment'. When I left the hospital that Wednesday, the Christmas holidays had not yet started, and I decided to go and say goodbye to my ex-classmates. I spent Thursday getting my bearings, and on Friday morning I walked across the road to the school as if nothing had happened. I dutifully attended all my classes – although I couldn't follow what the teachers were saying, having missed more than a month of the syllabus. I saw my classmates, answered their questions (yes, I'd had my hair cut…), wrote down a few mobile phone numbers, copied some notes from the lessons I had missed, and saw my teachers. Some of them suggested I prepare for tests the following term, and I nodded, smiling warmly and thinking to myself that it was just as well I was leaving.

Mum made an appointment with the headmistress of a boarding school, and three days later I was accepted there as a pupil.

I joined my new class – accompanied by the headmistress – at the beginning of January, right in the middle of the school year. You often read about this sort of thing in books, but it is quite different when you experience it first hand. All eyes were fixed on me, studying my every gesture while I stood there hardly daring to move. In the meantime, the smiling and unflappable headmistress explained to both pupils and teacher that I would be spending the rest of the school year with them. Believe me it was far more daunting than it sounds! After being introduced, I went and sat down at the only free desk, at the front of the class. I was given such a warm welcome and was so well cared for that I had almost no trouble catching up. Also, I had 30 new friends I could count on, and above all two guardian angels, Audrey and Léa, who patiently helped me.

Actually, going to a new school halfway through the year isn't such a bad idea. Everyone is eager to befriend you and if you aren't in very good shape it's even better because they all want to make a fuss of you. People were always asking me, 'Are you all right Mathilde?' I found this particularly touching and would cheerfully reply, 'Yes, I'm fine, thank you!' However, it can become irritating when 10 people ask you the same question during one break period. And one day, when I had already said, 'I'm fine, thanks,' about a dozen times, a sweet, well-meaning and thoughtful friend called Quentin asked me how I was, and I hit the roof! Everyone was shocked because I am usually so calm, but we all ended up laughing. Poor Quentin never dared ask me the fatal question again!

As far as eating is concerned I must admit I continued having problems for quite a while. I ate very little to begin with, alternating 'normal' phases with difficult phases. I still felt slightly disgusted by food and the fact is I only had 15 minutes to eat lunch because I had Latin class between

12.00 and 2pm followed by my session with the psychotherapist. And yet I had to accustom this tiny stomach of mine to eating again. Having to bolt down my food really didn't help and I suffered from terrible stomach cramps.

But I had made up my mind to be cured, and by the end of two months I no longer had to force myself to eat at all! My stomach cramps slowly went away, and my appetite came back to the point where I was having second helpings at every meal. By the summer everything was back to normal.

I remember one day going with Mum and some of my brothers and sisters and two aunts to eat ice cream – proper sundaes like the ones you see in films, covered in whipped cream, chocolate sauce and chopped almonds! In short, very filling. We all ordered one, and after a while Marc and Maguelone said they were full. I had already eaten mine and, despite having just had lunch, I finished both of theirs too!

As for my continuing treatment, I had a weekly appointment with a psychiatrist. These sessions helped me a lot. Every Tuesday I had to give a report on my progress. It was not easy to turn up without any baggage, and I had to admit when I hadn't eaten or was spending too much time on my own. I needed to convince her at all costs to stop my antidepressant! However, it is extremely difficult to hide your problems from a psychiatrist. I couldn't deceive her. I really had to be getting better!

And so I forced myself to laugh and joke with the others, to be sociable. The hardest part was 'letting go'. I felt out of practice, somehow it didn't seem 'natural'. But above all I was scared to open myself up completely. I still wanted to shield myself. I did spend a lot of time on my own. It is so much easier than having to externalise all the time, and I found boarding school tiring enough already. There really is no recipe for opening up. It just takes courage. You need to let go, not hold on. And this is precisely what I was afraid of: not having anything to hold onto.

A year later, in December, I was doing much better on every level. I started seeing a psychologist called Jeanne Siaud-Facchin. 'There's still a lot of work to do here,' she told me. With her I felt obliged to acknowledge my weaknesses, my lack of self-confidence, my pride. When you leave hospital everything goes brilliantly, but once the initial excitement has worn off, and you have to face reality, carry on with everyday life, the little problems begin to creep back.

We identified my weak points and tried to find solutions together, not just me on my own. I was forced to look at things I didn't want to see: Jeanne tugged on some painful threads in order to unravel all my knots. And, as with the psychiatrist, there was no way I could deceive her...

But the thing that most concerned me throughout my convalescence was the anti-depressant pills. If I was cured I shouldn't need them, and yet the psychiatrist continued prescribing them as though I was never going to get better. This undermined me. I took the tablets every evening, but psychologically I rejected them in the same way I had rejected food. In particular, the feeling that my progress was not down to me but to those pills was intolerable.

Moreover, I had a big problem with the anti-depressants: they affected my memory. My thoughts floated in a sort of mist, and I had difficulty finding my words and remembering people's first names (which is very annoying when you arrive at a new school and have to learn over a hundred) not to mention my lessons. It was difficult to make progress psychologically under these conditions, or even just to catch up at school.

I had not been taking the pills regularly for a while, and during the Christmas holidays just after I had started seeing Jeanne, I decided to stop taking them altogether. I refrained from telling the psychiatrist, and waited two weeks before telling my parents so they could see for themselves that I was all right. I felt liberated, like I had when the dentist took off my brace. I felt truly well, and had a new enthusiasm for life. This was a fresh challenge. Having said this, I wouldn't advise anyone on medication to do what I did and stop taking it suddenly because it can be dangerous.

Today I am doing really well. I am still a boarder, and in my final year at school. I hardly ever think about that period of my life. No more than anyone thinks about when they were 14. It is just part of my life. Still, I don't believe in referring to a past event as 'past history' until the people who witnessed it are no longer alive to tell the tale. For those living witnesses it will always be meaningful, and therefore linked to the present.

Similarly I never say that 'I have buried' that part of my life. No. I haven't buried it. On the contrary, I have placed it in the showcase of my memories, where it forms an integral part of my personal history; it is my way of refusing to accept that it served no purpose. To bury it would be to doom it to oblivion, and I can't bring myself to do that. I don't want others to go through the anguish, despair – madness even – that I went through. I suppose in a way I want to take revenge on the depression.

The only way I can express myself is through writing – hence this book. I wanted to tell other people who suffer from depression, You can live! To show parents what it is really like, and to say to everyone else, Look at the people around you, the future of some of them depends on whether you show indifference or kindness.

When I have finished school I would like to study medicine. Who knows, maybe I will become a psychiatrist.

# Afterword

## by Jeanne Siaud-Facchin

I was struck by the power and accuracy of Mathilde's words from the moment I began reading. Far from being a simple account, her book conveys the experience of depression with a raw sensibility and an extraordinary force. It is rare to gain entry into the intimate thoughts and feelings of an adolescent in this way, and with her book Mathilde has skilfully succeeded in 'bringing alive' her suffering so that other adolescents can recognise themselves and make sense of their own distress, and so that adults – and perhaps first and foremost parents – can better understand the drama played out in the private world of their depressive children. For everyone who feels powerless in the face of adolescent depression, Mathilde's account could prove more beneficial than any other form of explanation.

As a psychologist one encounters a great many cases of adolescent depression. Far too many. It is thought that this illness affects around 5 per cent of adolescents – twice as many girls as boys. More disturbingly, suicide is the second cause of death after road accidents among adolescents between the ages of 15 and 24.[1] It is a serious problem that requires specialised treatment, and as Mathilde learned to her detriment, mental health professionals are still very much in the dark where the special nature of adolescent mental illness, its treatment and care, are concerned. An increasing number of 'Adolescent Units' are coming into being in France – an initiative which appears to me both essential and unavoidable.

Depression is an aptly named illness in adolescents. It really is a time of *emptiness*; a time when they lose their footing, when the ground suddenly gives way beneath their feet and they feel as if they are being sucked into a void. They have the impression of being in the dark, of no longer existing, no longer knowing who they are or why they are alive. They desire nothing, and at times they crave everything – their craving is to fill this emptiness, this 'depression' in their lives.

Adolescent depression is unlike either childhood or adult depression. Indeed, I find it is almost regrettable to refer to such diverse pathologies by the same name. The main symptoms of depression in adults are mental anguish, guilt and an inability to face life, accompanied by a state of intense fatigue and a total loss of desire.

In children depression is multi-faceted: anxiety, aggression and hostility on the one hand, and on the other withdrawal, isolation, despair and insomnia or constant tiredness; together with numerous psychosomatic symptoms such as stomach pains, headaches and skin conditions... Indeed, it is possible that this multiplicity of

[1] *Les jeunes suicidants à l'hôpital*, Marie Choquet, Virginie Granboulan, Editions EDK, 2004.

symptoms results in a number of cases of childhood depression going undiagnosed.

Depression in adolescence is a true upheaval of seismic proportions which shakes all the foundations and certainties laid down during childhood. It was so nice and comforting being a child: believing your parents are all-powerful and can make everything better, believing things will get better, believing you can depend on adults, believing you can trust in life. And believing in magical things like Father Christmas, fairies and elves... even in the big bad wolf! At least the wolf is a comfortingly real manifestation of fear. And then adolescence rears its head, or, more precisely, puberty.

Adolescence is not a fixed state. It is a process of becoming, a transition. Etymologically speaking, the word *adolescent* means moving towards adulthood: *ad,* towards and *dulscere,* adult. I think it is dangerous to have crystallised what is essentially a process into a state, and ultimately into a marketing category. In today's society adolescence is no longer an experience one goes through, one *is* an adolescent. Referring to something as a *state* means being able to describe it, to define its common traits in terms of personality, attitudes and behaviour.

Adolescence in today's society imposes its own codes, codes Mathilde refused to accept. A way of dressing, of wearing certain brands, listening to particular types of music. And ways of behaving, of *having* to have friends, *having* to go round in groups, *having* to row with ones parents, slam doors etc... There is an implicit requirement 'You are an adolescent so you must behave like this.' We almost end up creating a new 'pathology' simply because adolescents who do not identify with this type of behaviour consider themselves 'abnormal'. Yet everyone has the adolescence that corresponds to them: it is engraved in their personal history, past, present and future, and the organising factor is personality. Adolescence is the conquest of psychological autonomy; what is at stake is the ability to become independent, to make decisions in life and accept the consequences, alone. The vulnerability of adolescents derives from this need to leave behind the emotional dependence of childhood. To move towards the frightening unknown and a future they are uncertain of measuring up to. In addition their sense of identity is still in flux: adolescents don't know what they want because they still don't know who they are. They are unsure of how to behave because they are a little like chameleons: their behaviour depends very much on other people's expectations, on which friend they are with at the time. Adolescents are 'unfinished'.

Recent neurobiological research has shown that the brain of the adolescent is not completely formed. Hitherto it was thought that the brain was fully developed by puberty, or around the age of 12, but it has now been discovered that everything still hangs in the balance for a good many years; the processes that regulate the emotions are not yet fully formed, and the system inhibiting and controlling behaviour situated in the frontal lobe of the brain is not fully functional. Adolescents seek emotional excitement without accurately being able to predict the consequences of their actions. The fondness for taking risks can also be understood in the light of neuroscience!

Adolescence is a time when everything constantly hangs in the balance: one has to choose and make decisions, to accept oneself as a boy or as a girl, to go through the ordeal of seduction, relationship with the other, sexual relations, and finally love. And love is not so simple because it means exposing oneself to possible suffering. Indeed, the universal plea of the adolescent could be summed up by the words, Tell me you love me!

Adolescence is a violent storm where you lose sight of all the old reference points before being able to determine the new ones. In order to be able to survive this storm, not simply in one piece but well-equipped to face the future, one thing is essential: a solid, positive self-image. So that even when the storm is raging one keeps one's footing, one is able to stay upright. Adolescents succumb to depression, as I said before, when they lose their footing completely, when there is nothing for them to hold onto, nothing with which to steady themselves in order to be able to carry on.

Anorexic episodes often indicate a difficulty with accepting one's body – or rather one's body-image – in adolescence. Anorexia is a markedly female symptom of depression, rarely affecting boys. It arises from a deep questioning of one's inner being. What stage am I at? Can I accept or cope with my body being desirable? Can I even accept that I might be looked at or, worse still, that a boy, a man almost, might desire me, might desire sexual relations with me? Anorexia is the fear of becoming, and of accepting, oneself – an immense fear. Mathilde's wish to disappear is a constant cry throughout her book. I don't believe that anorexia is an illness in its own right. For me anorexia indicates the path we must follow in order to help the adolescent in distress. Anorexia informs us as to the nature of the illness; it is a vital sign the adolescent leaves for us, and our job is to try to interpret it as quickly as possible in order to be able to intervene rapidly and effectively.

Mathilde's case was slightly different too, and slightly more complex – at any rate, no attempt was made to understand this difference. She refers to it discreetly in her book when she says, 'It's no fun being gifted!' For Mathilde is a gifted adolescent. Giftedness doesn't mean being cleverer than everyone else and finishing school aged 14 to become the pride and joy of your parents. Of course it means possessing a prodigious and versatile intelligence, but above all one that is *qualitatively* very different. Current neurological research confirms that gifted individuals think, reason, analyse and understand in very specific ways. Presented with a problem they will activate different areas in their brains, and in different ways, to other people in order to try to solve it. Specifically, their thought patterns are tree-like in structure and their cognitions (thoughts) move simultaneously in different directions at very high speeds. Their brains are constantly working: a question never leads to an answer but to another question, *ad infinitum*, and this complicates matters during adolescence, which is already a time of questioning. Gifted adolescents can never be certain of anything. Their acutely analytical minds continually taking in everything around them is a considerable hindrance when it comes to making choices. What to choose and why? Gifted adolescents are aware of too many things at once, and as a result are constantly analysing every element and possible outcome. It is exhausting.

In addition to their already extremely acute perceptive powers, gifted people possess a highly developed sensory capacity: they see things others cannot see, hear things others will never hear, and perceive things which are, on the whole, imperceptible...

Perhaps most importantly, gifted people are also hypersensitive and highly emotionally responsive: they are essentially emotional beings, constantly tuned into the emotional aspect of the world around them, and aware of other people's feelings sometimes to an intolerable degree. This is a weakening factor in their psychological development. It is painful to feel things too strongly, and one tends to try to protect oneself against it, particularly in relationships. Gifted people often have trouble forming relationships. They feel out of place, unusual, different without really understanding why. Gifted adolescents express this feeling very clearly: even with their closest friends they are conscious of a distance. They never feel a true sense of 'togetherness' with others, of completely fitting in. They also describe the three-dimensional way in which they experience everyday situations in life: 1) they observe the scene that 2) they are in the process of experiencing, and 3) they analyse it. Their brains are constantly working with an extraordinary degree of intellectual and emotional lucidity.

Extreme intelligence is a double-edged sword: it causes suffering and yet, ironically, nobody would ever think of sympathising with the sufferer!

So when a gifted adolescent breaks down and depression takes root, the main aim becomes to stop thinking, to stop activating that infernal thinking machine, the source of so much suffering, of so many painful emotions and endless questions. It is essential to consider all of these characteristics in order to be able to offer this type of adolescent the treatment he or she needs. Giftedness is not an illness but when it coincides with depressive disorder it takes on particular characteristics. Ignoring them is to run the risk of failing to provide the necessary treatment and support.

These characteristics are constantly in evidence throughout Mathilde's writing, in her choice of words and in the way she draws us in to her story, in her extreme thoughts and her heightened sensitivity. We realise just how often she felt misunderstood, alone and lost, infuriated by all the mistakes, all the incoherencies she couldn't help but be aware of, by all the diagnostic indecision and hesitation surrounding the treatment she should have received. And in the end the most crucial aspect of her personality was left aside.

Nevertheless, thanks to her remarkable inner strength Mathilde managed to pull through: giftedness also means possessing the possibility of infinite inner resources. Her book contains an important message of hope: one can go through unbearable suffering, and be unable to envisage the future, and yet emerge the other side with a renewed vitality that is stronger than despair. A true desire to live, fully.

This capacity to survive illness and be 'reborn' is common to all adolescents; giftedness only exacerbates its characteristics. Contrary to received opinion not everything is played out in adolescence. Adolescents are dealt a new hand from a new pack: people can experience a troubled childhood and an uneventful adolescence or go through a painful adolescence to become well-adjusted adults. Adolescence is like an avenue of hope opening onto the future.

Finally, for me this story is also the story of an encounter between a therapist and a patient, a psychologist and an adolescent, between Mathilde and myself. I have always found the idea of 'following' a patient's progress amusing, as if one walked along behind one's patients and allowed them to face the dangers of the world alone. I prefer the idea of a therapist and a patient sharing time, ideas and thoughts; attempting together to understand, unravel, re-examine, and re-work everything that is painful, complex, and confusing. The therapist's job is to give the patient the means to face life and feel good about their life. This is the experience Mathilde and I had. Therapy consists of two equally committed people working together in a constantly interactive, dynamic way.

Each new meeting with a patient is a challenge: one needs to update one's resources, to avoid digging in one place in search of an improbable source of illness but rather to attempt to draw out the healthy part that exists in all of us, even in the most severe stages of illness, and to use this as a basis from which to pick up again, to rebuild, together.

Therapy with adolescents must be conceived as a partnership based on mutual trust and respect. One must believe in adolescents in order for them to be able to believe in themselves, know how to identify and draw out their strengths, learn how to see them so that they can rediscover their own image, connect with them so they can reconnect with their own lives. Therapy with the adolescent is a complex human experience, but one that is enriching and full of potential and hope for the future.

It is essential in adolescence to find a motivating force in life. This vital energy, this will to live, is something all adolescents possess. We as adults must never turn our backs on them.

# About the Author

Mathilde Monaque was born in Brest, France in 1989. She developed severe depression at the age of 14. She is the eldest in a family of six and now lives in Bordeaux.

Jeanne Siaud-Facchin, author of the afterword to this book, is a clinical psychologist. After several years working in child and adolescent psychiatry at the Pitié-Salpêtrière Hospital in Paris and then at the Timone Hospital in Marseille, she founded, in Marseille, the first centre in France to specialise in learning difficulties (Centre CogitoZ) with a special unit for gifted children and adolescents. She has published two books and is currently recognised as one of the leading experts on the subject of gifted children.